Reduce BLOOD PRESSURE *Through* WEIGHT TRAINING

Ronald Deblois, BSc, BPE

Copyright © 2013 Ronald Deblois, BSc, BPE
All rights reserved.

ISBN: 148254069X
ISBN 13: 9781482540697
Library of Congress Control Number: 2013903453
CreateSpace Independent Publishing Platform
North Charleston, South Carolina

Contents

Disclaimer v

Medical Checkup vii

Acknowledgments ix

Dedication xi

Preface xiii

Introduction xvii

Section A: Physiology of Vascularization 1
    Chapter 1:   Fundamentals of the Circulatory System 3
    Chapter 2:   Effect of Cardiovascular Exercise on the Circulatory System: Vascularization 13
    Chapter 3:   The Physiology Behind Vascularization 19
    Chapter 4:   Cardiovascular Physiology in More Depth 23

Section B: Impact of Weight Training on Blood Pressure 27
    Chapter 5:   Weight Training Combined with Endurance Training 29
    Chapter 6:   Taking Your Blood Pressure and Mean Arterial Pressure 33

Section C: Adherence to the Program ... 37
    Chapter 7:   Challenging Current Practices and Concepts ... 39
    Chapter 8:   At What Pace? ... 47

Section D: Muscle-Fat Composition and Nutrition ... 51
    Chapter 9:   Fats in Your Diet ... 53
    Chapter 10:   Muscle versus Fat ... 61
    Chapter 11:   More Tips on Nutrition ... 65

Section E: Weight-Training Principles ... 69
    Chapter 12:   Basic Weight-Training Principles and Definitions ... 71
    Chapter 13:   Training the Whole Muscle ... 79
    Chapter 14:   Dimensions of Muscle-Initiated Movement ... 87

Section F: Fitness Programs ... 91
Part 1: Types of Fitness Programs ... 93
    Chapter 15:   Choosing a Fitness Program for a Specific Sport ... 95
    Chapter 16:   Choosing a Fitness Program for Health and Quality of Life ... 99

Part 2: Personal Fitness Program ... 105
    Chapter 17:   My Personal Fitness Program ... 107
    Chapter 18:   Is Your Program Working? and Afterthoughts ... 127

Appendix A: My Personal Research Record: Interpretation and Assessment ... 129

Appendix B: One-Sitting Readings from November 26TH, 2010 ... 133

References ... 137

Suggested Readings ... 141

Index ... 143

DISCLAIMER

I do not provide safety guidelines for the weight-training exercises I recommend in this book. For this purpose, please employ the services of a *certified* trainer in the initial stages of your program.

Medical Checkup

Regardless of your age, please get a medical checkup prior to beginning a fitness program, especially if you are on medication. A proper fitness program requires strenuous effort on your part, especially in the later stages. If you suffer from an insidious illness, such as high blood pressure, your program may trigger a severe, life-threatening event. Tell your doctor what you are planning to do so he or she can give you a proper evaluation.

Acknowledgments

Many thanks to Jeanne Cote, a graduate of the Ontario College of Art in Toronto, Canada, for patiently producing the excellent illustrations found in this book.

Dedication

I am honored to dedicate this book to the memory of a loving father, Gerry de Blois, as fine an example of integrity and the work ethic a son could possibly hope to have.

Preface

Articles often warn that hypertension, the main risk factor for cardiovascular disease, afflicts one in four adults in North America. The following information sheds even more light on the severity of the situation. In 2000, nearly one billion people, or about 26 percent of the world's adult population, had hypertension. The *Canadian Medical Association Journal* reported that rates of hypertension were up 77 percent between 1994 and 2005. These rates are still rising because nothing tried so far has worked. For example, refer to the following guidelines recommended to the public by the Public Health Agency of Canada:

1. Be active two and a half hours a week to achieve health benefits.
2. Focus on moderate to vigorous aerobic activity throughout each week, broken into sessions of ten minutes or more.
3. Get stronger by adding activities that target your muscles and bones at least two days per week.

These guidelines are too general to be effective, and very few people heed this advice. There are no suggestions for *monitoring progress*, which is vital for success.

Current medical treatments for cardiovascular problems are mostly palliative (that is, not cures): none of the technological treatments for heart disease, such as balloon angioplasty, thrombolytic therapy (clot-busting drugs), antiarrhythmic drugs, pacemakers, or the new "renal denervation" technique, can slow the buildup of fatty deposits in arteries. This process, known as *atherosclerosis*, causes one's blood pressure to rise. *Reduce Blood Pressure through Weight Training* is a medication-free lifestyle tool that will allow millions to avoid these drastic medical interventions by offsetting atherosclerosis and other causes of hypertension through vascularization: the addition of capillaries to organs stressed by exercise (Chapter 2).

How do we vascularize? Currently, fitness experts recommend reducing or avoiding hypertension with cardiorespiratory endurance activities, but these activities really only vascularize the heart and lungs. This is certainly necessary, as it protects these vital organs that comprise about five pounds of the body's weight. At best, however, cardio reduces resting systolic pressure by about ten to fifteen points. *Reduce Blood Pressure through Weight Training* recommends adding its unique weight-training principles to one's exercise program to vascularize a large percentage of the body's seventy pounds or more of skeletal muscle, reducing blood pressure by much more (Chapter 5). Six hours or fewer of reasonable effort per week should reduce it by *fifty points or more*. That's marvelous, and this is not even a twenty-hour-per-week, exhaustive bodybuilding program; neither are bodybuilder weights needed! Assume that person A reaches muscular exhaustion (failure) at ten repetitions while lifting a maximum of twenty pounds for an exercise, whereas person B is stronger and reaches the same point with fifty pounds. By reaching failure, both vascularize *the same percentage* of the stressed muscle in spite of their difference in strength.

Note also that, because a woman's hormone balance differs from a man's, weight training does not cause women to become muscular (bulk up) like a male. Female bodybuilders do bulk up—intentionally—because they tend to work out twenty or more hours per week. They also dehydrate themselves to stand out in competition. In this program's six hours or so per week, a woman will enjoy the benefits of weight training and its improved toning, with minimum bulk.

Inactivity is harmful to your health!

Adequate intensity and long-term adherence are required for success. To help you stay with the program for months, you can use five simple yet reliable tests to monitor your improvement to determine if you should increase—*or decrease*—intensity. Senseless, Rocky Balboa–style effort will only cause you to quit the program early. Using the

Progressive Overload Principle (Chapter 12) and the Principle of Moderation (Chapter 17), you will acquire, safely and *at a reasonable pace*, a tolerance for the physical discomfort that will produce the desired anatomical changes. These principles will also show older participants that they are quite capable of more intensity than they thought possible. Watered-down programs do not work. My own experience is proof: I am over seventy-three as I write this and still work with greater intensity than most subfifty participants for a reasonable six hours or fewer per week, with a one-week respite every six weeks or so.

Being properly informed also encourages you to continue your workouts. This is why the opening chapters (1 to 3) explain clearly the process of vascularization and its importance for reducing resting blood pressure. More advanced physiological principles explain further why vascularized muscle mass reduces blood pressure (Chapters 4 to 6).

I also explain why body mass index and skinfold techniques (Chapter 7) justify a complete reliance on a unique waist-weight procedure (Chapter 10) for keeping track of muscle-fat composition. You will see why you should increase your muscle mass, with its higher metabolic rate, *by five to fifteen pounds or more.*

I explain how to use nutritional guidelines and proper diet along with your weight-training program (Chapters 9 and 11). Dieting alone causes you to lose much-needed muscle mass—not just fat.

Understanding how to train *"the whole muscle"* is critical to your success. The more muscle mass you vascularize, the more your blood pressure will drop (Chapter 13). You also need to know how to measure blood pressure over multiple readings (Chapter 6).

Learning how to distinguish between a sports-oriented program versus a health-oriented one (Chapters 15 and 16) will give you a better perspective on your objectives. A comprehensive health-oriented program not only controls blood pressure, but also improves strength and offers protection against osteoporosis, along with numerous other fitness benefits (Chapter 16). You can adapt the program provided by this book to the equipment and facilities at your disposal.

Reduce Blood Pressure through Weight Training gives you the ability to better judge the validity of faddish fitness programs offered by gym instructors and the confusing and irrelevant fitness information in the media. You will no longer be at the mercy of their jargon (much of which is simply incorrect).

INTRODUCTION

The numbers are chiseled into my memory: 320/180, a staggering level of hypertension. Imagine my shock and grief when I learned that Gerry, my father, a once-bustling, industrious, good-natured fifty-six-year-old man apparently in the best of health, had suffered a massive stroke. He could no longer speak and dragged the right side of his body like a heavy, cumbersome anchor.

Before and after the stroke in 1971, his five-foot-nine-inch frame weighed a deceptively ideal 160 pounds. According to his surgeon, a clot had completely plugged the small opening remaining in his left carotid artery; it had narrowed severely over the years with cholesterol. This cut off the blood supply to the left side of his brain, the part that controls the right side of the body, essentially starving it to death. My father passed away in 1990, after a bedridden three years: terminating a gruelling, vacuous life.

After his stroke, his doctor explained to my brother and me, then in our early thirties, that we had a good chance of suffering the same fate. He suggested strongly that we not smoke and that we maintain a healthy weight; at the time, neither was a problem for us. Yet his suggestions did not mention physical activity. The doctor's prediction held true for my brother, whose most strenuous activities following graduation were golf and pickup hockey until the day he went into a coma at the age of sixty-two in 2003. Two blood clots had entered his brain. Three or four days later, he was disconnected from life support.

Fortunately for me, I had had a passion for weight training starting in high school, initially because I played football. And I never stopped working out. Partly that was because I became a physical education teacher—but I also did it for the personal challenge. I'd developed a healthy tolerance for intense training. "The weights" felt good. At the time, weight training was considered good for functionality, but nobody (including myself) seemed to connect it with cardiovascular health.

Because of my family history, I had always checked my blood pressure periodically, and it had always been fine. In fact, I began to notice over the last eight years that, oddly enough, my blood pressure readings—diastolic as well as systolic—were decreasing somewhat. Was that because I had retired and had been working harder in the gym? Then in 2007, at age sixty-seven, I hurt my shoulder in September and was required by my physiotherapist to train much less and at a lower intensity until the end of January 2008, after which I was allowed to again start increasing my effort. Less than two weeks later, on February 8, I had a routine annual physical and was dismayed by my blood pressure readings. They were 190/78 and 172/90. It appeared that without proper weight-training effort my inherited propensity for high blood pressure had surfaced. Duly, I was prescribed a low daily dose of Lisinopril (10 mgs). At the time I also purchased a blood-pressure monitor that could upload readings to my computer and calculate the average of any sequence of readings. As I gradually increased my workout intensity, I read my blood pressure regularly. The results intrigued me so much that the subject became my research project. My monitor's capabilities became important. I've provided my readings (more than 12,500 from February 2008 to October 2011), as monthly averages with a corresponding analysis in the appendices at the end of this book.

Although my discovery of a relationship between weight training and blood pressure is what really prompted me to write *Reduce Blood Pressure through Weight Training*, many other factors influenced my decision:

- Teaching health and physical education for many years sensitized me to our society's health concerns.

- From what I have observed in the gyms I have worked at, I believe that far too many people start fitness programs with the best of intentions but quit prematurely. This is usually because they either work too hard at the outset or have absolutely no idea whether their program is helping them.

- Equally worrisome is that many follow programs that are of low benefit because they don't work intensely enough.

- Many never even come to the gym because they are intimidated by a lack of understanding of basic fitness principles.

If we could get all of these people to follow an effective program, the preventive health benefits would reduce our health-care costs significantly, and the fitter individual would be much happier, more autonomous, and therefore less of a burden on society.

It is also worth repeating that the fitness industry is rife with jargon, fads, and gimmicks that do nothing better than confuse and mislead the beginners, not to mention waste their financial resources. *Reduce Blood Pressure through Weight Training* should provide the insights needed to wade through this maze of unreliable information to allow anyone to choose a valid fitness program to achieve his or her desired goals.

Somewhat in the same vein, I feel that currently, most doctors' advice on exercise is too sketchy to be helpful. I might even suggest that this book, much like regular medication, be prescribed to all patients at risk of cardiovascular problems. Doctors around the world are now being asked to put more emphasis on *prevention* in their practice.

My main objective as a physical education teacher was always to encourage my students to embark—for life—on a physical fitness program aimed at improving their health and quality of life. I always felt it was my duty to stress what would provide the greatest good for our society and for my students. I may have retired, but I haven't changed my philosophy—only its target demographic. I hope that the information in this book will help you avoid the pitfalls mentioned above and persuade you to include a proper fitness program in your life.

Section A:
Physiology of Vascularization

CHAPTER 1

FUNDAMENTALS OF THE CIRCULATORY SYSTEM

The body is such a great organism. Provide it with the appropriate activity, and it will reward you by changing itself in ways that improve your life immensely. Many of these wondrous changes take place in the circulatory system.

Each of your organs (skeletal muscles, liver, heart, brain, intestines, and so on) is permeated and nourished by its own bed of copious capillaries that allow blood to access *all parts* of the organ. Simply put, each of these capillary networks receives oxygenated (red) blood from an artery, while, at the opposite end, the network is drained by a vein that returns the now-used (blue) blood to the heart. The blood then goes on to the lungs for reoxygenation.

Capillary Beds and Blood Flow

Capillary beds exist in every organ in the body.
A few are labelled below.

Arrows indicate the direction of blood flow.

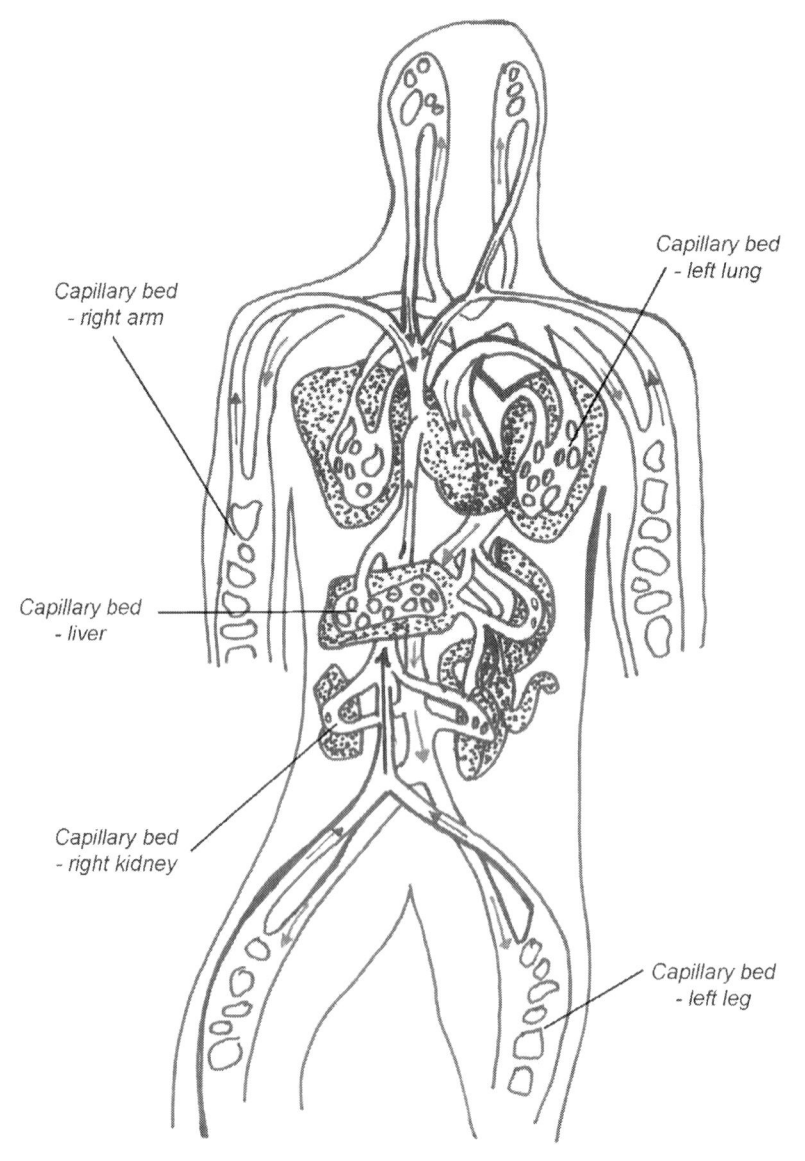

Capillary bed - right arm

Capillary bed - left lung

Capillary bed - liver

Capillary bed - right kidney

Capillary bed - left leg

Task - colour arrows in the arteries red
- colour arrows in the veins blue.

CHAPTER 1

Arteries have thick walls of smooth muscle tissue that contract to help push blood away from the heart and toward the capillary beds. They eventually branch into smaller blood vessels with muscular walls called arterioles that will direct the incoming blood into the capillaries. The arteriole walls have the capacity to *vasoconstrict*—to reduce the size of their internal diameter—thereby reducing the amount of blood they will deliver to the capillaries they are connected to. They can also *vasodilate*—that is, relax to allow their diameter to increase—to allow more blood to pass on to the capillaries they are connected to. They do this in response to metabolite levels in the blood—waste or end products of metabolic processes in the body.

Capillary walls are very thin, one-cell-thick membranes that allow the exchange of nourishment and waste products at the molecular level between the organ and its blood supply (e.g., when oxygen from the blood replaces the metabolite carbon dioxide within the organ's tissues). This exchange cannot take place in arteries or veins because of their thicker muscular walls (although a vein's walls are somewhat thinner than an artery's).

Unidirectional valves inside the veins help maintain blood flow, largely against gravity, toward the heart. Because of the superior compliance properties of veins—their ability to stretch—about 60 percent of the body's total blood volume is usually held in the venous system at any given moment.

The circulatory system delivers oxygen (among other things) to each organ and prevents the buildup of waste products, such as the metabolite lactic acid, as much as possible. Lactic acid—also known as fatigue acid—can gradually impede an organ's function. A sprinter running at top speed produces lactic acid in working muscles much faster than the circulatory and respiratory systems can break it down. After about sixty yards or so, the excessive buildup of lactic acid within the leg muscles will cause the sprinter to slow down *involuntarily*. If he continues, within ten seconds the same leg muscles will be saturated with lactic acid and stop contracting against the runner's will, forcing a stop. Once stopped, his breathing will be labored in an attempt to inhale as much air (oxygen) as possible to clear the excess lactic acid from the worked muscles. (A jogger undergoes the very same process; it simply takes longer to get to the slowdown and stop due to the lower running speed. The circulatory and respiratory systems can cope better with the slower rate of production of lactic acid.)

An aside: In fact, though, lactic acid might not necessarily be the culprit. Over the last seven or so years, many research hypotheses have suggested alternative mechanisms. Because the biochemistry underpinning these changes is quite complex, however, the conclusions are not yet firm. One suggestion is that lactic acid quickly breaks down into the substrate lactate and hydrogen ions; the ions increase acidity (reduce the pH) within the working muscle and contribute to the pain and fatigue. Whatever the details, the runner decelerates and eventually stops, and we know that increasing oxygen in the working muscles reverses the problem. And increased vascularization (Chapter 2) helps increase the availability of oxygen to the muscles.

Your Resting Pulse Rate

The pulse rate (heart rate) is the number of times the heart contracts, or beats, per minute. Your resting pulse rate is a reliable baseline reading because it is always taken under the same conditions: while your body is fully rested. It is best taken in the sitting position, say, thirty minutes or so after you get up in the morning, rather than later in the day when lactic acid has accumulated within the body. (The sitting position is the standard because prone or standing positions give different results.) Before taking your pulse, give your heart a few minutes to calm down after you sit.

General Procedure: Turn your left hand palm-side up. Place the first two fingers of your right hand along the outer edge of your left wrist just below where your wrist and thumb meet. Slide your fingers toward the center of your wrist until they feel the tendon. Press down with your fingers until you feel the pulsation. Count the number of beats for one minute. Do not use your thumb instead of your two fingers because it has its own pulse. This could provide a false result.

The more cardiovascular training you do, the more your resting pulse rate will *go down* over time. The further it is below seventy-two—the resting pulse rate of the average human being—the better. Marathon runners, because of their intensive training, have resting pulse rates of forty beats or less per minute. For the average person, reducing the resting pulse rate of a healthy heart to fifty or sixty beats per minute might be enough to significantly reduce the risk of cardiovascular disease, assuming a concomitant blood pressure decrease. Take your resting pulse rate three or four times a week to see if your fitness program is working. If it does not go down, increase the intensity of your workouts, but only in small increments.

How important an indicator of cardiovascular health is your resting pulse rate? Italian researchers found that having a resting pulse rate above seventy beats per minute increases your risk of dying of heart disease by at least 78 percent.

Understanding Blood Pressure and Hypertension

Please refer to the following cross-sectional diagram of the heart if need be when its parts or functions are mentioned throughout the book. Notice that the muscular wall of the left ventricle is much thicker than the right ventricle's wall because it must push blood through the whole body and eventually back to the heart when it contracts. The right ventricle only sends blood a short distance to the lungs and back.

Blood Flow through the heart's chambers

Arrows below indicate the direction blood follows as it flows through the heart.

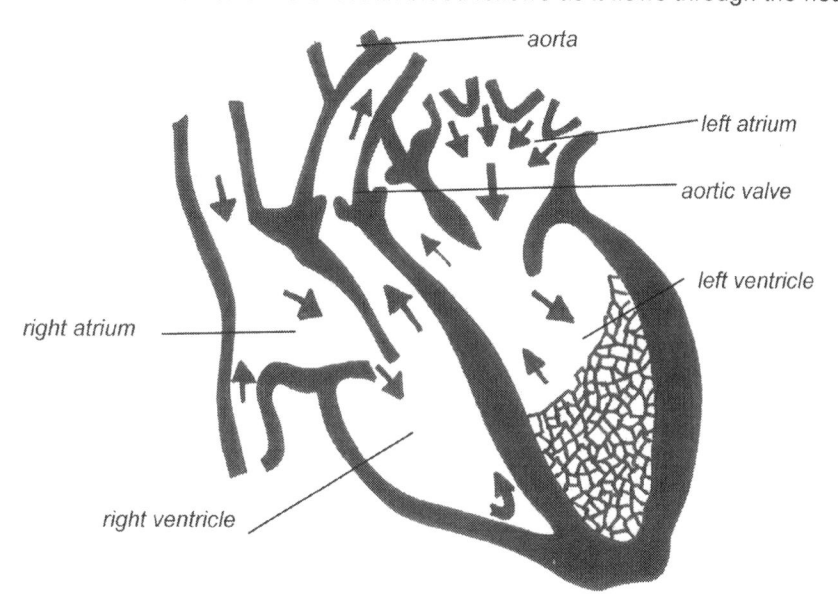

- aorta
- left atrium
- aortic valve
- left ventricle
- right atrium
- right ventricle

For the body to survive and function properly, blood must flow through the circulatory system *at a rate fast enough* not only to nourish its tissues adequately, but also to prevent the excessive accumulation of waste products constantly being produced in the organs.

In other words, to meet the body's metabolic needs (at rest or under stress), the heart and aorta must contract alternately (The Windkessel Effect, Chapter 4) with a force *strong enough* to cause the blood to flow steadily at this critical rate.

Blood pressure is always expressed, with systolic pressure as the first number, in a ratio format; diastolic pressure is the other (as in a systolic/diastolic pressure of 115/75). Systolic pr*essure* is the measure of the force of contraction of the heart's left ventricle. Diastolic pressure is a measure of the aorta's force of contraction: a recoil force exerted by the aorta's wall against the distending blood it received from the left ventricle that just contracted. This recoil occurs between heartbeats, during the heart's relaxation or diastolic phase (The Windkessel Effect, Chapter 4). Without this well-timed force, blood would flow more slowly through the circulatory system and in a pulsatile fashion, because it would pause momentarily between heartbeats. The purpose of this force, therefore, is to allow a continuous stream of blood to flow smoothly and efficiently through the circulatory system at the mandatory flow rate dictated *by the body's metabolic needs*. Without the aorta's contribution, systolic pressure would increase significantly and possibly to harmful levels, because the heart would have to contract harder to compensate for the reduced, less efficient flow rate.

The maximum recommended pressure while the body is fully rested is 115/75 or lower; it used to be 120/80. Today, readings between 115/75 and 150/90 are considered prehypertensive and requiring medical scrutiny because of the increased risk for cardiovascular disease. Pressure readings chronically at or above 150/90 are considered hypertensive and potentially detrimental to cardiovascular health.

Increased resistance to the movement of blood through vessels can reduce its flow rate. If it falls below the rate that meets the body's metabolic needs, blood pressure has to intensify to compensate: both the heart and the aorta have to contract with greater force. The following factors can cause risky increases in resistance:

- *Atherosclerosis.* All internal surfaces of the circulatory system, including the heart, are lined with a very important tissue composed of a single layer of large, flat cells. This tissue is called the endothelium. Because blood is a viscous (thick and sticky) fluid, its movement through vessels exerts a shear stress on this endothelial layer: a force that wants to drag it along with the flow. This constant shear stress often produces small lesions (tears) in the fragile endothelium, especially during episodes of increased blood pressure and near areas where large arteries fork off. The blood usually heals these lesions, although, unfortunately, some can develop into pathogenic sites that reduce the size of the artery's lumen (its internal passageway) as plaque composed largely of fatty acids such as triglycerides and LDL cholesterol accumulates within the lesion. Atherosclerosis is the name given to this condition of plaque build-up. Now, halving a lumen's radius increases resistance to blood flow a colossal sixteenfold. Blood pressure rises proportionately, further increasing shear stress on the endothelial layer and the possibility of atherosclerosis, especially in individuals with high cholesterol levels.

Atherosclerosis

As illustrated in the following diagrams, atherosclerosis is a gradual narrowing of passages (lumen) within arteries as a result of fatty substances (plaque) being deposited inside the artery. Cholesterol is the main culprit.

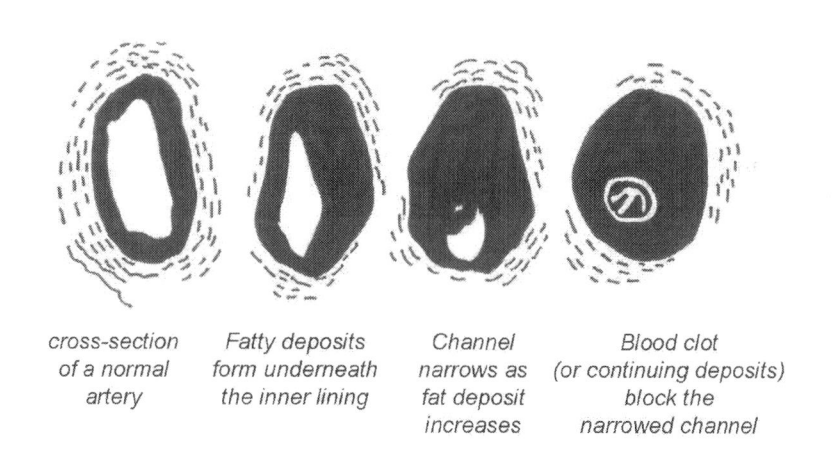

| cross-section of a normal artery | Fatty deposits form underneath the inner lining | Channel narrows as fat deposit increases | Blood clot (or continuing deposits) block the narrowed channel |

- *Arteriosclerosis* is a hardening of artery walls, which is especially dangerous when it happens in the aorta. The atherosclerotic plaque and/or the muscular wall tend to harden and lose elasticity, possibly through calcification, age, or other factors. The artery wall becomes rigid and therefore incapable of stretching adequately in response to the outward pressure of blood flowing through its lumen. Resistance to blood flow increases in addition to the resistance created by the narrowing of the internal diameter of arteries through plaque formation (atherosclerosis). As a rule, the older we get, the more inflexible our arteries become.

- A sedentary lifestyle. This degrades the efficiency of your cardiorespiratory system by reducing the number of capillaries in each organ (hence the total cross-sectional area available for blood flow). This detraining effect is explained in Chapter 2.

There is more to share on atherosclerosis. An atherosclerotic site can also progress into a blockage that closes a blood vessel and causes tissues beyond to die from lack of nourishment. Just as ominous, an atherosclerotic site can release a dangerous blood clot that can be carried downstream to block another narrower blood vessel, again cutting off tissue nutrition. Occasionally, blood pressure is high enough to rupture fragile capillaries, causing blood to seep into intercellular spaces, clot, and starve the cells they surround. The consequences of these necrotic events depend on the extent (from negligible to significant) and location of the damage. In the heart, they cause heart attacks; in the brain, they cause strokes. (Keep in mind that damaged brain cells do not regenerate.) Other vital organs are also at risk for devastating results: liver, kidneys, lungs, and so on.

Both systolic pressure and diastolic pressure increase in direct proportion to a higher resistance to blood flow, which can cause blood pressure to attain higher, possibly prehypertensive or greater, levels. Remember that symptoms of hypertension are often imperceptible and therefore insidious: it is the silent killer. This is why you should measure your resting blood pressure regularly at the pharmacy or, even better, at home (Chapter 6). Once a year at the doctor's office is probably not enough, especially if you are over forty-five years old. I also strongly recommend frequent checks to monitor the *effectiveness of your fitness program.*

The *Journal of the American Medical Association* (*JAMA*) said in 2011 that, for some age groups, the risk of cardiovascular disease *doubles* with every increment in blood pressure of 20/10 above 115/75. Although lack of exercise or poor dietary habits can lead to dangerous hypertension, many other neurological and physiological causes can raise blood pressure. Regardless of the cause, a significant increase in blood pressure definitely means a visit to the doctor. Although exercise reduces resting pulse rate and helps control blood pressure, please understand that a low resting pulse rate does not necessarily guarantee a low resting blood pressure. You should monitor both regularly as you progress through your fitness program.

Without hesitation, I would say that the most important objective of your fitness program is to control, as effectively as possible, your arterial blood pressure. The next chapter explains how a properly planned exercise program does this through vascularization.

CHAPTER 2

EFFECT OF CARDIOVASCULAR EXERCISE ON THE CIRCULATORY SYSTEM: VASCULARIZATION

The anatomical and physiological changes I describe below are called the "training effect" or vascularization. We achieve them through a long-term, low-intensity cardiovascular exercise program, such as running two miles outdoors (or running indoors on a treadmill) three or four times a week—a practice most health experts recommend. The first change mentioned is an increase in capillary density.

Improving Capillary Density

A properly designed cardiovascular program increases the number of capillaries in exercised organs—their capillary density (Chapter 3)—while the number of *arteries and veins* servicing each of these organs remain the same. For example, jogging essentially stresses and thereby increases the capillary density of the heart, lungs, and, to a minor extent, leg muscles.

Important: These improvements in capillary density are created by temporary intense increases in metabolic needs through short or extended bouts of exercise stress, whereas the body's at-rest metabolic needs do not change. Why? Referring to the legs only, cardio activities fundamentally do not increase the size of these stressed muscles because the individual's body weight is a resistance—opposition to movement initiated by skeletal muscles—that varies little during this type of activity. Muscles increase in size (hypertrophy or bulk up) only in response to increases in resistance (Chapter 12). Losing body fat represents a decrease in resistance. As you progress through this book the importance of understanding these distinctions will become clear.

Following are some of the benefits resulting from the added capillaries:

- Each extra capillary gives added protection by providing an alternate blood-flow route within an organ should any vessel be blocked by clots or atherosclerosis. This is especially beneficial in vital organs such as the heart and lungs.

- Capillary beds, with their numerous capillaries, allow huge amounts of material to enter and leave the blood because they maximize the area across which exchange occurs while decreasing travel distance to target tissues. More capillaries through vascularization augment this efficiency, so that the metabolic needs of the vascularized organ at rest are now *more than met*. Because the body always tries to maintain homeostasis—that is, a stable physiological state—it will have to reduce supply to meet the organ's unchanged demand at rest. To do this, its arterioles must then vasoconstrict (Chapter 1) in order to slow blood flow through the organ. However, for smooth blood flow through the body, flow rate between the heart and the constricted arterioles cannot be faster than the now-diminished flow rate through the trained organ's capillary bed. Through feedback, the heart and the aorta must decrease this rate (heart to arterioles) by reducing their force of contraction accordingly. In fact, both events—vasoconstriction of the arterioles and reduction of the contractile forces of the heart and aorta—must happen *simultaneously*. This has the welcome effect of reducing the individual's systolic and diastolic blood pressure at rest and in response to stress.

The addition of capillaries to the organ's network also reduces its internal resistance (Chapter 4), causing blood to flow even more rapidly through the organ. The arterioles, heart, and aorta react to the organ's surplus nourishment just as they do in the above case. This reduces resting and stress blood pressure further.

Additional Changes

Cardiovascular training has other benefits for the whole body in addition to the organs being stressed:

- Reducing the mass of fat tissue (resulting in less passive body weight to support) through cardio exercises reduces the body's metabolic needs. Less demand on the heart, the aorta, and the rest of the circulatory system means a welcome reduction in both systolic and diastolic blood pressure, at rest and under conditions of stress.

- Current research seems to indicate that LDL ("lousy") cholesterol actually exists in the form of large and small molecules, with the small molecules being responsible for creating the damage that leads to cardiovascular disease. Conclusions from such research indicate that exercise reduces the blood's number of small LDL cholesterol molecules while increasing its content of large, innocuous LDL molecules. This reduces the possibility of atherosclerosis and the formation of blood clots within the blood vessels and, thus, the possibility of increased resistance to the flow of blood over time. Hypertension is kept in check. (HDL, "happy" cholesterol, simply put, was thought to reduce the possibility of atherosclerosis by cleaning excess LDL cholesterol from the arteries. Proper exercise was thought to further increase protection against atherosclerosis by augmenting the level of HDL in the blood. Much to the chagrin of researchers, it has recently been shown that increased levels of HDL cholesterol do not reduce the occurrence of cardiovascular disease.)

- Increasing the lumen diameter of arteries allows a higher volume of blood flow and decreased resistance (Chapter 1). This means that the same flow rate can occur at a reduced velocity, lessening the force required from the heart and the aorta. Doubling its size, if this was possible, would reduce its resistance to blood flow by a factor of sixteen.

- Cardio exercise increases the blood's red-cell count. This means that the blood can deliver the same amount of oxygen at a reduced velocity through vessels. This would lower blood pressure.

- Each muscle cell (cardiac, smooth, and skeletal) is powered by its mitochondrion, small organelles found within the cells that generate the energy they require to perform their many functions. Adequate exercise increases the mitochondrial content of each stressed cell, allowing it to contract more efficiently and with greater power when needed. Mitochondria use glucose in combination with oxygen to generate their power. This should provide a quicker response to the need for muscular power.

- Exercise prevents hardening of the arteries by maintaining their flexibility longer, reducing resistance to blood flow.

- Lung efficiency improves. The lungs exchange oxygen and carbon dioxide faster, which also improves blood pressure.

- Blood circulates more efficiently. Well-functioning muscles have a "milking" action, squeezing their own veins every time they contract. This rhythmic mechanism assists blood flow through the veins' unidirectional valves back toward the heart.

- Endothelial lesions are *less likely*. Reductions in blood pressure decrease flow velocity and shear stress within vessels, reducing the probability of endothelial lesions that could lead to the formation of pathogenic atherosclerotic sites.

The cumulative impact of these changes will certainly have a significant positive impact on the blood pressure of an individual. The potential is enormous! Chapter 4 provides a few more possibilities.

Going forward, I use the term vascularization to refer to the sum of the above changes. Improved vascularization of the organs through a well-chosen fitness program causes the circulatory system to respond more effectively to the metabolic needs of the body. Consequently, pulse rate and blood pressure go down, proportionately and chronically.

Remember that each blood pressure reduction of 20/10 will halve your risk of cardiovascular disease.

Exercise is believed to force organs to vascularize through adequate stress—almost as if an organ says to itself, "I must deal with this periodical misery by preparing myself for it," and expands its capillary bed so that (among other things) it is always on call to help alleviate the discomfort of any physical or emotional stress. The nice thing about this is that the extra capillaries also help to reduce blood pressure while someone is at rest.

Conversely, abandoning a training program leads to a *detraining effect*—a reversal of any vascularization gains. Previously trained organs lose capillaries, increase resistance, and reduce blood flow, proportionately raising blood pressure—not a desirable outcome! Remember that halving the cross-sectional surface available for blood flow increases resistance sixteenfold.

Postexercise Hypotension

Exercise has a separate impact on the individual's well-being. Blood pressure rises during exercise, but biochemical mechanisms dampen the effect so that it doesn't rise to dangerous levels. This effect remains after termination of the exercise to cause blood pressure to remain below normal levels for about four to twelve hours after exercise (this is postexercise hypotension). If you work out three times per week, your possible thirty hours a week of hypotension may improve the long-term health of your cardiovascular system by reducing *further* the probability of vessel lesions.

CHAPTER 3

THE PHYSIOLOGY BEHIND VASCULARIZATION

Vascularization is mainly about increasing an organ's capillary density through exercise stress. This chapter suggests two interrelated physiological processes that might contribute to this objective. As you are reading about the two studies that explore these processes, please keep in mind that the physical activities used in these experiments duplicate *very closely* the exercises proposed in this book.

Firstly, anaerobic and aerobic processes are responsible for producing energy to meet the body's needs. When energy is produced in the *absence* of oxygen, it has been produced anaerobically, whereas production is aerobic when oxygen is required. The primary source of energy for a dynamic resistance activity such as weight lifting is anaerobic (Fleck and Kraemer, 1987; Fox and Mathews, 1974). In part, this is because dynamic resistance has a static component; it is also due to the sometimes high intensity and short duration of the exercise. However, dynamic resistance activity does use aerobic energy, proportional to the number of weight-lifting repetitions (reps) per set and the duration (number of sets) in a workout. (Increasing the weight lifted would probably have a similar impact.)

For example, the oxygen *requirement* of five sets (six to twelve reps each) of supine leg presses by a group of untrained males is charted in Fig. 4.6 (Tesch et al., 1990) shown below. The chart shows that oxygen requirement gradually rises over the first three sets, then stabilizes for the remaining two.

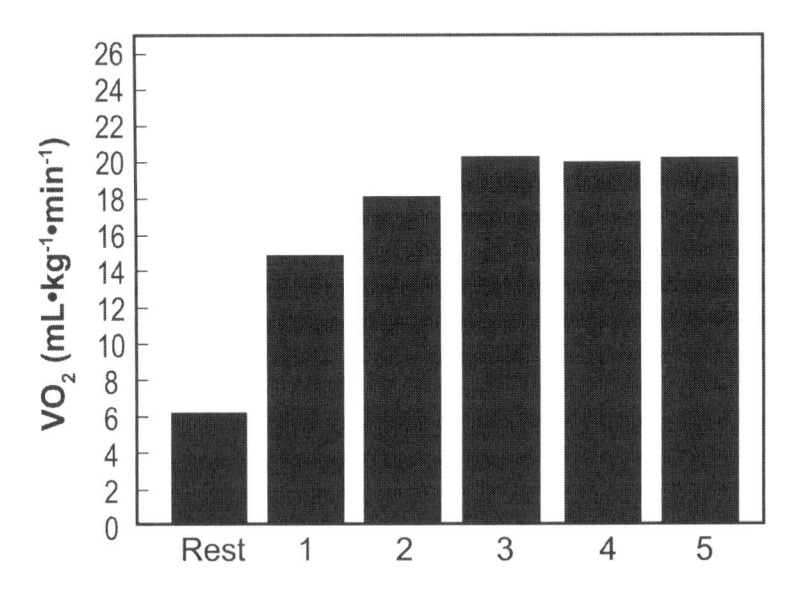

FIGURE 4.6. Aerobic Contribution to Dynamic Resistance Exercise
Oxygen consumption was measured before and during five sets of 6-12 repetitions of supine leg presses. The values represent the combined results of two groups: one performed only the concentric (lifting) phase, and the other performed both the concentric and eccentric (lowering) phases. The addition of the eccentric phase represented such a low additional energy cost above just the concentric energy expenditure that it was not separated out.
Source: Based on Tesch, P. A., P. Buchanan, & G. A. Dudley: An approach to counteracting long-term microgravity-induced muscle atrophy. *The Physiologist.* 33(Suppl. 1):S-77-S-79 (1990).

This study clearly demonstrates that weight training uses oxygen to produce some of the energy it requires, at least to the tune of approximately 33 to 47 percent of the average maximal oxygen consumption (VO2 max) for the subjects involved in *this* study. VO2 max is a measure of *the maximum volume* of oxygen per unit of time an individual's body can transport and process during a strenuous exercise. The higher the individual's VO2 max, the better his or her fitness level. Does this need for oxygen stress the circulatory system enough to improve capillary density within the muscles used, as it does for cardiovascular training? The next study provides the answer.

From a second study, Peter Krustup, Ylva Hellsen, and Jena Bangsbo published a paper in 2004 on an interval-training experiment indicating that intense intermittent resistance exercise (interval training) causes a stressed muscle's capillary bed to expand. Six healthy, habitually active male subjects performed dynamic, one-legged, knee-extensor exercises using the quadriceps on an ergometer while in the supine position, three to five times per week for seven weeks. At an intensity corresponding to about *150 percent of thigh VO2 peak*, there were fifteen sets of one-minute bouts, separated by three-minute rest periods; *exhaustion* (failure in this book) by the end of each session was intended. While one thigh was exercised, the other was used as a control for comparison.

The study clearly demonstrated that capillary density *increased significantly* within the trained thigh. The number of capillaries in contact with each muscle fiber increased by 19 percent for slow-twitch fibers and 21 percent for fast-twitch fibers. Slow-twitch fibers improve a muscle's endurance, whereas fast-twitch fibers give it more power. In addition, the greater number of capillaries may have elevated microcirculatory blood volume in the trained muscle. A possible explanation for the increase in blood flow at the high workloads is that the approximately 5 percent increase in muscle mass and 20 percent gain of capillaries in the trained leg expanded the microvascular volume at the onset of exercise.

Author's comment: These major changes occurred after only seven weeks of controlled activity. Imagine the changes *after months and years* of using similar exercises. (Brachial [at the arm] blood pressure was not taken during this experiment.)

Note: There was no reference to mitochondrion, described in Chapter 2, in either of the above studies. However, when oxygen is available (aerobic), each of these organelles is capable of creating twenty times more energy per glucose molecule than it can in the absence of oxygen (anaerobic). The quality of the oxygen-delivery system is therefore an important factor with regard to the effective operation of the body's muscles.

CHAPTER 4

CARDIOVASCULAR PHYSIOLOGY IN MORE DEPTH

Why Adding Capillaries Reduces Resistance and Blood Pressure

The individual capillaries that form a parallel network within an organ essentially have *identical resistance* to blood flow. It has been determined that the overall resistance of the network within the complete organ is equal to the resistance of an individual capillary **R** divided by the number **n** of parallel capillaries found in the network: in other words, overall resistance to blood flow within an organ can be expressed by the ratio **R/n.**

So the more the parallel elements within the network of an organ, the lower its overall resistance. This means that adding capillaries to the network of any single organ through exercise reduces proportionately its internal resistance to blood flow. If cardiac pressure and aortic pressure remained the same, blood flow through the organ would greatly increase, but as we've seen (Chapter 2), the heart and the aorta must reduce their force of contraction to match the organ's metabolic needs, and hence reduce resting systolic and diastolic blood pressure. This means that the more organs a fitness program vascularizes, the more significant the impact on overall blood pressure and cardiovascular health, during rest and physical and emotional stress.

Contraction Pattern of the Heart

The heart diagram in Chapter 1 delineates the path of blood through the heart, but does not show *the order* of the heart's contractions. It does not follow the sequence of right atrium, right ventricle, left atrium, and left ventricle implied by the diagram; in fact, *the two atria* contract together, simultaneously filling their respective relaxed ventricles with blood. Once done, they both relax and remain relaxed while *both ventricles* contract in unison (systole) to push their contents out into their designated arteries. Both ventricles then relax together so they can simultaneously be filled by the blood flowing freely through the open valves of the relaxed atria. Eventually, simultaneous contractions of the two atria *top up* the ventricles. This pattern—simultaneous contraction of the two atria followed by the combined contraction of the two ventricles—repeats itself, producing the individual's pulse rate.

Relaxation of the Ventricles

Following systole, the ventricles relax by means of a calcium-releasing mechanism in their myocardial muscle cells. This relaxation period is called *diastole*. Pressure eventually drops to *zero* within these chambers, producing a pressure gradient between them and their respective atria, where the blood's pressure, at the end of its long trek through the body and lungs, is now down to 2 to 4 mmHg. Millimeters of Hg (mercury) is a measure of the amount of force needed to raise a column of mercury the stated height. Consequently, during diastole, blood flows from the point of *highest* pressure (atrial chambers) to the point of *lowest* pressure (ventricular chambers) to refill the ventricles. This pressure difference is what allows the blood to constantly continue to flow.

The Windkessel Effect

The Windkessel effect describes the aorta's contribution to the efficient flow of blood through the circulatory system. Let us begin its series of events with a systolic contraction by the heart's ventricles.

During the heart's systolic phase, contraction of the left ventricle pushes a fraction (stroke volume) of the blood it contains through the aortic valve into the aorta. Beyond the aortic valve, this incoming blood comes up against blood that is moving in the same direction (downstream), but more *slowly* than itself. The incoming blood thus piles up against the slower-moving, outgoing blood. This piling up causes the aorta, due to its natural compliance (ability to stretch), to *bulge out* around its full circumference into the shape of an elongated doughnut.

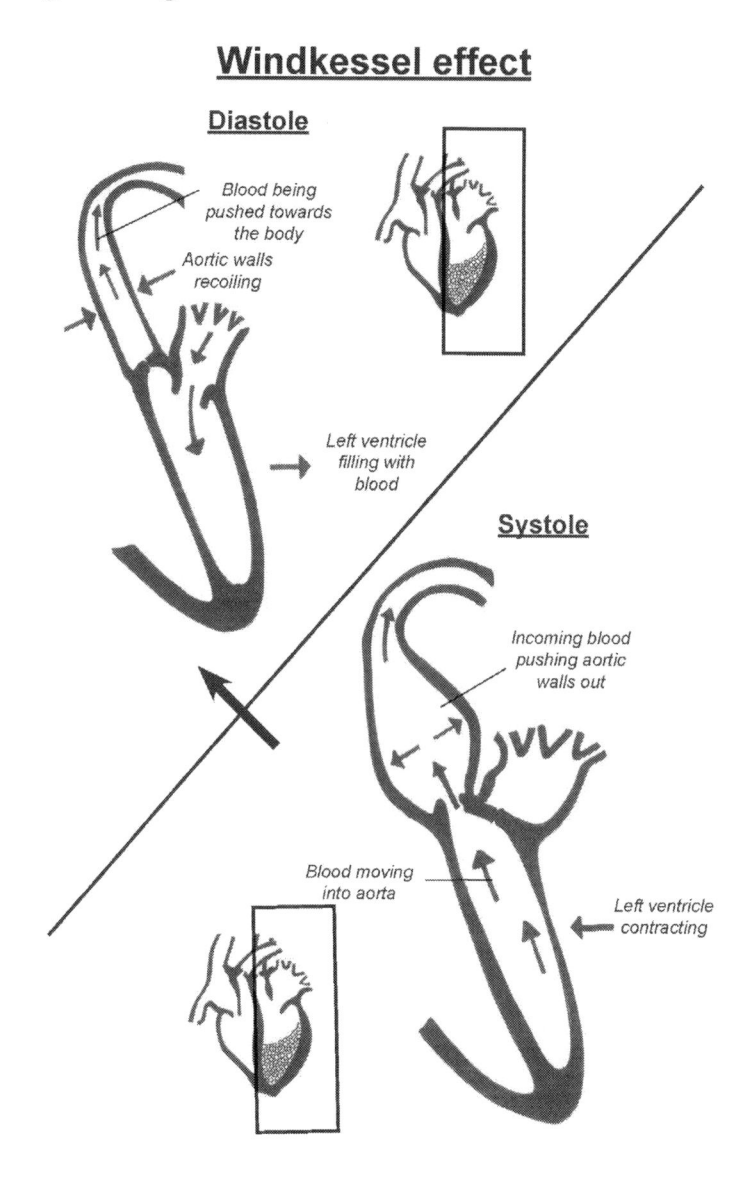

Windkessel effect

Diastole

- Blood being pushed towards the body
- Aortic walls recoiling
- Left ventricle filling with blood

Systole

- Incoming blood pushing aortic walls out
- Blood moving into aorta
- Left ventricle contracting

25

This situation continues until the ventricular contraction ceases and the heart enters its diastolic or resting phase. During this phase, due to a stretch reflex, the aorta's wall *recoils* back to its original shape. The pressure from this action *closes* the aortic valve and pushes forcefully on the blood that initially deformed the aorta, causing it to move downstream toward the body. This prevents blood flow from hesitating momentarily between beats during the heart's resting phase. The blood's flow through the circulatory system is therefore faster and smoother, as opposed to pulsatile and slower.

The force exerted between heartbeats by the aorta's walls on its engorging blood is referred to as *diastolic pressure*. (Although the aorta is the main contributor, diastolic pressure is in fact the end result of all the forces exerted by all the arteries between the aortic valve and the brachial [arm] blood pressure cuff while blood pressure is being taken. As a shortcut, I use the term "aorta" to mean all these arteries.)

Note that the neurogenic and biochemical feedback mechanisms that control the strength of contraction of the heart's cardiac tissue (systolic pressure) also control the strength of contraction of artery walls including the aorta (diastolic pressure). Coming from a *vascularized organ*, these same feedback signals will therefore reduce diastolic as well as systolic blood pressure. The more vascularized the organ, the lower the blood pressure. (See Appendixes A and B for practical examples that demonstrate just how efficient these mechanisms can become.)

Section B:

Impact of Weight Training on Blood Pressure

CHAPTER 5

WEIGHT TRAINING COMBINED WITH ENDURANCE TRAINING

Although cardiovascular endurance training has a positive influence on the health of your circulatory system, for results that are more potent, you should combine it with weight training. Let's explore why.

We call the blood vessels of the heart and lungs the *core* of the circulatory system, and the vessels that deliver blood from the heart and through the body its *peripheral* part. Most peripheral vessels pass through skeletal muscles, which comprise about 35 percent of the body's weight.

So, why weight train? Currently, fitness experts recommend that people control blood pressure using only cardiorespiratory endurance exercises, but these activities essentially only vascularize the heart and lungs. Cardio certainly improves function in and protects these two vital organs. However because the heart weighs about one pound and the lungs four pounds, the best they can do for blood pressure is to lower systolic pressure by about ten to fifteen points, since they only reduce core resistance to blood flow.

An innovative approach using effective weight-training principles vascularizes skeletal muscle mass (Chapter 3), decreasing peripheral resistance to blood flow. Since skeletal muscle mass represents about seventy pounds of an average person's 165-pound weight, or *fourteen times* the combined mass of the heart and lungs, vascularizing it can potentially reduce systolic pressure by an additional 140 points. Fat tissue cannot be vascularized.

My research has shown that five or six hours of reasonable effort per week—possibly less—should be enough to reduce systolic pressure by *fifty or more points*, and diastolic pressure by *thirty or more points*, depending on an individual's effort (see Appendix A). This certainly means many fewer lesions in the endothelium over the course of a lifetime, and hence a significant decrease in the probability of atherosclerosis!

The more skeletal muscle a person vascularizes adequately—especially the large muscle groups of the body (back, chest, shoulders, legs)—the better the effect on blood pressure than if he or she only vascularized the heart and lungs. This is best done with a weight-training program that is intense enough: for some of your weight-training sets, you must push yourself to failure to saturate the stressed muscle with lactic acid. This is what stimulates vascularization. *Failure* means that you continue your reps until you cannot do even one more. Chapters 12 and 13 provide additional weight-training principles that can also help vascularize muscle mass very effectively.

Adding weight training to your program offers other advantages. It burns more calories, leading to fat loss and a further reduction in your blood pressure! A major objective of this program is to increase your body's muscle mass by *five to fifteen pounds* or more, which will improve your functionality, but, at the same time, muscle tissue has a significantly higher metabolic rate than fat tissue. This means it burns more calories whether you are moving or at rest—promoting more fat loss. Combined with a proper diet that further reduces your body-fat percentage, your blood pressure should go down even more.

This should convince you that your fitness program should include both cardiovascular and strength training components for best results.

Muscle Hypertrophy and Blood Pressure

Chapter 2 explained how cardiovascular training can reduce overall blood pressure. We assumed, largely for ease of comprehension, that the exercise program did not change the size of the trained organs (such as the leg muscles). Some readers may be concerned by the fact that weight training can *hypertrophy* stressed muscles (i.e., make them larger) because it seems to them that the increased mass would raise the body's metabolic needs, increasing demand on the heart and aorta, and thus would *raise* blood pressure. That would be true, were it not for the fact that the 5 percent or so increase in muscle mass also vascularizes, through *angiogenesis*—the development of new blood vessels from pre-existing vessels. That is, the new muscle tissue also develops new blood vessels, keeping up in capillary density with the original part of the trained muscle. At the very least, the reductive impact on the individual's blood pressure will be the same as if the muscle had not hypertrophied. (Note that *the reverse process would occur with a loss of muscle mass*.)

It may also be that because the complete hypertrophied muscle now contains substantially more parallel capillaries, its overall resistance (**R/n,** Chapter 4) may decrease considerably, because as its capillary resistance (**R**) remains constant, its **n** increases significantly. In other words, **R** is divided by a much larger **n** value, and blood therefore flows with an even greater velocity through the *larger* muscle (the original mass plus the 5 percent new mass) than if the extra mass had not been created. It is therefore fair to assume that the extra mass of hypertrophy could reduce systolic and diastolic pressure even further, in spite of the concomitant increase in the body's resting metabolic need. It could mean that the more skeletal muscle you build, the more you will lower your blood pressure. Hopefully these comments will spur a researcher's curiosity.

CHAPTER 6

TAKING YOUR BLOOD PRESSURE AND MEAN ARTERIAL PRESSURE

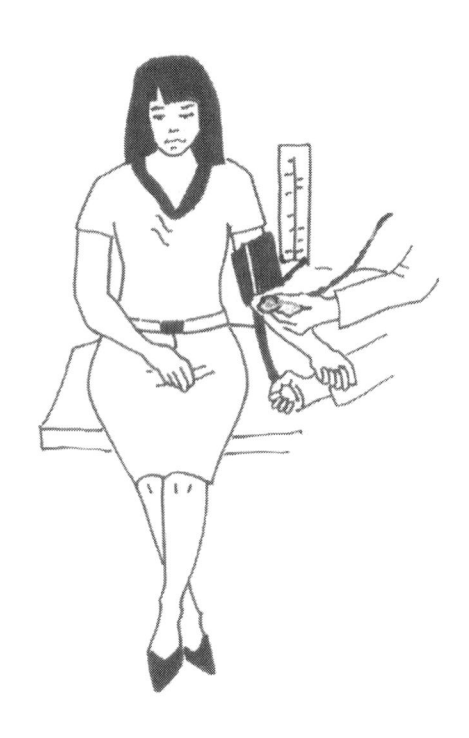

Like your resting pulse rate, your resting systolic and resting diastolic blood pressure should go down in response to an appropriate fitness program. The best way to verify that it does is by taking your resting blood pressure frequently. Doing it *at rest* is important, because that is when your blood pressure is lowest; it gives you a reliable baseline with which to compare *future* at-rest readings as you progress through your fitness program.

You must be fully rested and as stress-free as you can be. Your environment should be at a comfortable room temperature, and you should not be hungry. Sit motionless and wear loose, non-restrictive clothing, with your back against a support. Morning is best, because fatigue, physical effort, and emotions (positive or negative) throughout the day cause your blood pressure to fluctuate. You should wait half an hour or so to measure blood pressure after eating or being active.

A stressful situation, whether physical or emotional, might raise your systolic pressure by sixty points. If, at rest, you're normally at the recommended reading of 115/75, a temporary rise to 175 is relatively benign. But if your resting systolic pressure is chronically 150, the same stressful situation could raise your systolic pressure to 210. A reading of 150 is already bad enough, but 210 is even more likely to damage the interior walls of your arteries and lead to atherosclerosis. Awareness of your baseline reference value should encourage you to take the precautions necessary to avoid dangerously high levels of blood pressure, especially in response to stress.

For greater reliability and better understanding, you should take multiple readings at each sitting. Forty or more times per session is more valid than a single reading that may give you the wrong impression (e.g too low). Seeing how systolic and diastolic measurements can vary over forty or more readings gives you valuable insight into your circulatory system's response to varying conditions. You should then calculate the average of your readings. (For this purpose, I recommend the iHealth app if you have an iPhone; it can store all of your readings.) Changing averages, rather than single values that might be high or low, are *better indicators* of how effectively your fitness regimen is affecting your cardiovascular health. (Single elevated systolic and diastolic values taken at rest, however, cannot be ignored, as they might signal bad news.) With the iHealth app, you can delete values that are invalidated because you coughed, the phone rang, somebody walked in, and so on, since they would skew the average. If you start too soon after you've been active, your initial readings will be elevated but succeeding readings will eventually stabilize. The early ones can then be deleted.

Mean Arterial Pressure and Driving Pressure

For a more accurate picture of the relationship between systolic pressure and diastolic pressure, let's consider an example. Assume your resting blood pressure measures 115/75. This means that during one full heartbeat, the pressure at a certain point in the brachial artery of the arm ranged from a systolic high of 115 to a diastolic low of 75. If pressure had descended gradually and evenly from 115 to 75 during the heartbeat, the average blood pressure for the heartbeat would therefore be (115 + 75) ÷ 2 = 95 mmHg.

However, the pressure does not go down gradually and evenly here: it has been determined that the systolic interval accounts for only 20 percent of a heartbeat's duration, whereas the diastolic lasts the remaining 80 percent. To compensate for this, doctors put more emphasis on diastolic pressure by using the following formula when they calculate *mean arterial pressure* (MAP), which more truly represents the "driving pressure" required to push the blood around the entire circulatory system:

MAP at rest: MAP = $\frac{1}{3}$(SP - DP) + DP
SP = systolic pressure and DP = diastolic pressure.

So for the measurement 115/75, MAP = $\frac{1}{3}$(115 - 75) + 75 = 88 mmHg. The result is down by 7 from the 95 obtained when blood pressure was assumed to go down gradually from 115 to 75. This suggests that a lower diastolic pressure may have a greater protective effect for the individual than we might otherwise assume.

But again, single elevated systolic readings taken at rest can be serious indicators of cardiovascular health, despite their occupation of only 20 percent of a heartbeat's time.

Section C:

Adherence to the Program

CHAPTER 7

CHALLENGING CURRENT PRACTICES AND CONCEPTS

There are many know-it-alls in the gym. I will provide additional information that will allow you to hold your own against poorly founded criticism and advice, and you will better understand why you are doing what you are doing.

Body Mass Index and Skinfold Measurements

Muscle gain and fat loss are two major objectives of my program. For monitoring muscle-fat composition, I recommend the waist-weight technique explained in Chapter 10. Neither the traditional Body Mass Index (BMI) nor the skinfold measurements technique measure changes in muscle content; they only measure fat content, and even then, they are not adequate.

The *Body Mass Index* is a mathematical formula that divides your body mass by the square of your height. The result supposedly correlates strongly with the body's fat content. A BMI between twenty-five and thirty is considered overweight; above that, you are obese.

However, a high Body Mass Index can result just as well from high muscle mass as from fat tissue. This could therefore mislead a perfectly healthy individual (mesomorphic or muscular build as opposed to endomorphic, which implies being overweight) and possibly a large-boned individual to shed weight in the form of desirable muscle mass. Also, partly because muscle tissue is much denser (and heavier) than fat tissue, reliance on BMI in scientific studies could cause researchers to overstate rates of obesity in target populations.

On November 4, 2004, Dr. Salim Yusuf and his research team at McMaster University published their experimental discovery that waist-hip ratio measurements (Chapter 10) are at least *three times* more effective in predicting the risk of heart problems than BMI. In fact, his team found only slightly higher BMIs in heart-attack patients than in experimental control subjects representing the general population. Waist-hip ratio is more valid because, through the hip measurement, it allows more effectively for *muscularity*. The BMI, in my opinion, is vague and no better than a plain visual inspection.

Skin fold calipers

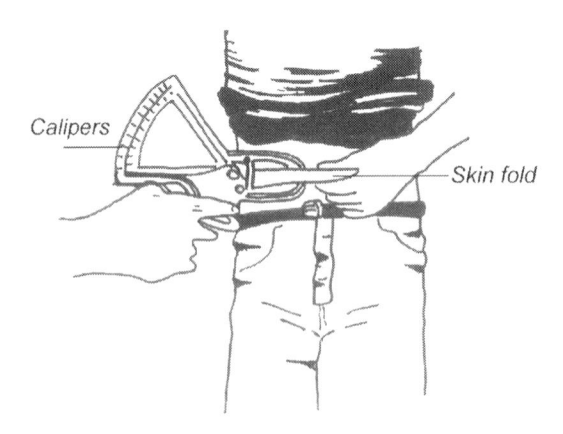

The *skinfold technique* is supposed to measure the distribution of fat around an individual's body. It is an indirect method that adds the thicknesses of five or so pinched skinfolds at different locations on the body and matches the total to a standardized table of body-fat composition. The skinfold method lacks *reliability*; it is difficult to duplicate the exact folds measured from one session to the next.

Aside from being unreliable and time-consuming, these fat-measuring methods are unnecessary.

As you work out, fat is reduced *equally* in all parts of the body, regardless of the exercise. For example, whether you work the triceps or do leg squats, you reduce fat content wherever it is stored, including the waist. Exercise is not *site-specific* for reduction of body fat. For this reason, a simple girth (waist) measurement shows whether an exercise and diet regimen actually provide the desired results. If your waist circumference decreases every day, fat has been lost without a doubt. Waist size goes down in direct proportion to fat loss from all over the body. The reverse is also true: an increased waist size means someone is fatter. You can adjust your exercise and/or diet program according to waist measurements alone. In fact, reducing abdominal fat (in particular, visceral fat, which is fat that surrounds your internal organs) should be a priority, as it is the most dangerous for raising the body's cholesterol level.

Muscular Endurance

Today's fitness and physiology publications do not correlate cardiovascular fitness with weight training. And physical education students are taught that weight training only develops strength and not cardiovascular endurance in the worked muscles. They are told that "muscular endurance," a nebulous quality resulting from the improved anaerobic capacity of the trained muscle, is responsible for the fact that *more repetitions* per set can be done with the same weight after extended training. The scientific studies from Chapter 3, however, provide significant support for the conclusion that increased aerobic capacity (through increased capillary density) supporting the augmented mitochondrial density of each cell is largely responsible for this fact.

Another theory is that slow-twitch muscle cells that have more endurance have replaced fast-twitch cells. This, however, only happens in response to long-term, low-intensity exercise, whereas weight training involves very short-term bursts of high-intensity exercises that tend to produce fast-twitch muscle cells with little endurance. Most of the extra repetitions, at the rate of *one or two per three or four weeks*, must therefore come from vascularization of the skeletal muscle being stressed. Oxygen can be transported to it at a significantly faster rate, allowing lactic acid accumulating during a set to be broken down more effectively.

Starting Weights

The best way to increase your risk of straining a muscle or pulling a tendon is to force them to lift a weight they are *not prepared for*. Many trainers and fitness publications suggest that your starting weights should be 60 percent of your maximum lift. but an untrained person should never try to lift his maximum, one-repetition weight for an exercise, especially at the *beginning* of a program. There is no rush to get into heavy weights. They can injure unprepared muscles, or tendons and ligaments which heal very slowly and interfere with your progress. Rather, start with a weight you have no difficulty lifting for twenty repetitions and, over the course of months, use the Progressive Overload Principle (Chapter 12) along with the Principle of Moderation (Chapter 17) to get to the heavier weights gradually and safely.

Weight Training and Hypertrophy of the Heart

Many fitness and health professionals see weight training as a static exercise that causes the heart to hypertrophy (chronically get larger and stronger). Let me explain why this is illogical.

Pernicious (harmful) hypertension involves strong, continuous contractions of the heart for twenty-four hours a day, seven days a week. This has been proven to cause significant chronic hypertrophy of the heart muscle—especially the hardworking left ventricle that must force blood to flow through the whole body—much like a skeletal muscle overloaded by a resistance (Chapter 12). For the heart, this is a pathological condition. Note that activities such as marathon running that stress the heart constantly for extended periods (four or five times per week during long laborious practices and competitions) might also cause the myocardium to hypertrophy.

Strength training, however, should only be considered static in isometric exercises: extended periods of maximum contraction against an immovable resistance. Isotonic weight-training exercises, on the other hand, are dynamic, because they involve moving a weight repeatedly and rhythmically through a specified range (e.g., bicep curls). Stressed muscles contract and relax during the exercise much like a leg muscle's action during jogging. Breathing is also rhythmical because, much like natural breathing, the lifter inhales as the stressed muscle contracts and exhales as the weight is returned to its starting position, during each repetition.

In lifting, the skeletal muscle pump (the "milking" action by the working muscle) helps blood circulate around the body. That is, the working muscles squeeze their own internal veins when they contract, and the one-way valves inside them ensure that their blood flows in one direction: toward the heart. These mechanisms (rhythmic movement, rhythmic breathing, and milking action) dampen somewhat the temporary, *exertion-induced* increase in blood pressure. Blood pressure rises significantly higher during *isometric* exercises because the supportive mechanisms are absent there.

To clarify further let us look, for example, at a weight-training set that goes to *failure* in twelve repetitions. Such a set lasts about thirty seconds (four reps per ten seconds). The first eight reps prefatigue the muscle by building up its lactic acid level to about the same degree as leg muscles that have sprinted more than eighty yards. The last four reps eventually *saturate* the muscle with so much lactic acid that it cannot do a thirteenth repetition. As soon as the set ends, lactic acid production ceases and the circulatory system begins to break down the accumulated amount quickly within the muscle. After two minutes, the muscle is partly back to normal, and labored breathing has stopped.

In this book's program, most of the twenty sets per two-hour session are taken to failure. This means that, at thirty seconds per set, only about ten minutes of tough exertion are required per two-hour session. That's *less than* thirty minutes per week if you do three sessions. Blood pressure will rise above normal during the lifting actions of the weight program, but not likely to extremes. These exercises are designed to use the blood-pressure-dampening mechanisms. It is highly unlikely that the contractile cardiac tissue will hypertrophy chronically in response to this level of stress.

In addition, in my program, the heart's myocardial capillary bed is expanded by the stress of three half-hour sessions of aerobic activity per week and weight training does the same for the skeletal muscles it stresses. Because of the efficiencies brought about by these core and peripheral vascularizations, the heart and aorta can meet the body's needs by contracting with less force during systole and diastole. Long-term consistent overloading does not occur, so neither the heart nor the aorta will get bigger in response to this regimen. In fact, the *weaker* contractions might actually cause cardiac tissue and the aorta's smooth muscle tissue to atrophy (Chapter 12) slightly over time. Hypertrophy of the heart does not take place here.

Heart Rates and Workout Intensity

Fitness books advocate different ways of using heart rate as a guide for choosing the initial and ongoing intensity levels of an exercise program's endurance component. These choices are *arbitrary and unreliable.* (For example, in the "heart rate reserve" method, the maximum heart rate target is defined as the arbitrary number 220 minus your age) I don't need to go into detail about any of these heart rate techniques; I offer a reliable alternative. There is a better way!

Be patient and start your endurance training at a very low intensity level (Chapter 8). Increase it gradually in keeping with the Progressive Overload Principle (Chapter 12). Keep using your resting pulse rate in conjunction with the other four tests suggested in this book as a guide for increasing or decreasing your program's intensity. Because you always take your pulse rate under the same, fully rested conditions, you can watch its behavior: it should go down gradually in response to a proper level of exercise intensity. I have noted that the average person at rest has a pulse rate of seventy-two beats per minute, but hypertension occurs frequently among such people. The further below that number your resting pulse rate is, the better.

An improving resting pulse rate, however, does not guarantee low blood pressure, the main objective of the fitness program. Be sure to take your resting blood pressure regularly. The longer you follow a program, the more aware you will be of what you have to do to create the changes in your circulatory system to reduce your resting pulse rate and blood pressure. Take your resting pulse rate three or four times per week for a better assessment and proper motivation. It only requires a few minutes of your time.

Perceived Exertion Scale

Some recommend the "perceived exertion scale" technique for choosing a fitness program's intensity level. It uses subjective levels of difficulty to identify the degree of exertion needed over the duration of a program:

- very, very light
- very light
- fairly light
- somewhat hard
- hard
- very hard
- extremely hard
- very, very hard

These subjective evaluations depend on many variables that may or may not provide valid results. How you feel is not reliable unless you are ill! Resting pulse rate and resting blood pressure give *concrete, conclusive results* that suggest changes in intensity levels much more reliably. You may need to increase your treadmill speed, run the same distance faster, or maybe even run and weight train less. Using your resting pulse rate is not to be confused with the heart rate techniques suggested in much fitness literature.

Battery of Tests

Many fitness professionals recommend a battery of performance tests to ascertain a client's fitness level, indicating the starting point for a fitness program and its intensity. They then retest to assess progress. The tests (walk-run, step-up tests, treadmill tests, etc.) are especially useless for the beginner who has been inactive for a long time. Maximum-effort tests only prove someone is out of shape; this, he or she already knows. Rather, people should start fitness programs patiently and at a very low intensity level and build up gradually (Chapter 8).

The five simple, yet very reliable tests I recommend (resting pulse rate, resting blood pressure, waist-weight measurements, and waist-hip ratio discussed in Chapter 18) more effectively measure the efficacy of a program as it proceeds, and are much less time-consuming. Performance improvements in the program's exercises also provide excellent feedback on its effectiveness.

Faddish Exercise Programs

Be wary of faddish exercise programs, especially those that imply that you can achieve your goals *without exertion*. "Swiss exercise balls" are a good example: lifting weights while sitting or lying on an inflated ball supposedly to strengthen your core muscles (abdominals and lower back). The problem is, because of the wobbly surface, you can only use lighter (and therefore less effective) weights for the targeted muscles. Traditional exercises on *stable* surfaces work the core muscles, yet you can use heavier, more effective weights to vascularize the targeted muscles. (And don't forget that you can always work the core muscles directly!) Just apply my tests to evaluate any new program easily.

CHAPTER 8

AT WHAT PACE?

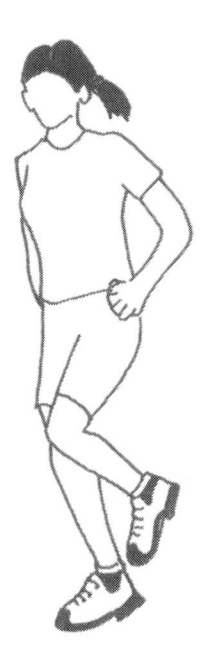

You wouldn't believe how often I see a novice come to the gym, suit up, warm up for a few minutes, then get on a treadmill and run at a punishing pace for an hour, sweat dripping from his nose and getting his T-shirt soaking wet. Obviously, he has finally made a firm decision to "get in shape." In *every* such case that I've observed, the individual lasted two or three weeks and was never seen in the gym again.

This is the "no pain, no gain" philosophy at work. You think you must push yourself to the point of pain—to the absolute limit—in every workout, if you hope to make any progress. In fact, this is the best way to discourage yourself from working out, simply because you will quickly condition yourself against your training regimen. Each new training day, consciously or subconsciously, you will dread going back to the gym, knowing that you will have to tolerate yet another bout of severe discomfort. This common Rocky Balboa approach should be avoided at all costs. "No pain, no gain" is a strong deterrent to the regular, long-term participation necessary for meeting real fitness objectives. Rather, *tolerance* for physical discomfort should very *gradually* improve to build up to the effort level that causes vascularization and other fitness benefits to take place. And guess what: the effort required is much less intense and much more reasonable than the one described above.

For example, for an unfit, inexperienced person, I recommend ramping up to an effective cardiovascular running program like this:

* Three times a week, walk four hundred yards per day at a normal pace, with at least a day's rest between each session.
* Two or three weeks later, increase the distance by two hundred yards every week or two, up to about one mile per day, three workouts per week.
* For the next two or three weeks, jog one hundred yards and walk the rest of the mile.
* The next two or three weeks, jog two hundred yards and walk the rest of the mile.
* Each couple of weeks, add one hundred yards until you can jog, with confidence, the full mile.
* After three or four weeks of jogging a full mile add two hundred yards every two or three weeks up to two miles, three times per week.
* Then, gradually reduce the time for this distance (that is, increase jogging speed), aiming to reduce resting pulse rate to sixty beats per minute or less.

For general fitness purposes, two miles (and possibly even less), three times per week, should be more than enough. You have so many choices: treadmill, swimming, cycling, cross-country skiing, and so on.

You can vary the approach depending on your fitness level. If this formula is too difficult, start even more slowly. Few physical changes occur in the early part of the program, but the important thing is that one should gradually and reasonably adapt to rising levels of effort that do produce the desired anatomical changes. Chapter 17 applies the same sensible, progressive method to the weight-training component of your fitness program.

I applied this reasonable approach as a teacher. At the time (and maybe even today), preparatory courses for physical education teachers recommended that on the first day of class, student fitness levels should be assessed by timing them in a one-mile run. Yet most young people are inactive over the summer unless involved in athletics. We did not need this kind of test to find out what we already knew. To avoid resentment and maintain positive attitudes, I used the more sensible approach of improving my students' fitness level gradually over the course of the year. I felt my students would be more likely to stick with physical activity over time.

Diminishing Returns

Another thing that discourages fitness is that people spend more time in the gym than they need to. This gets in the way of other interests, and can actually produce *diminishing returns*. Take my sample fitness plan above. By the time someone is jogging two miles three times a week for a couple of months, that person probably has vascularized about 80 percent of his or her five pounds of heart and lungs—close to optimal. Vascularizing the remaining 20 percent might require three or four times as much effort, but with little additional improvement to the cardiovascular system.

Diminishing returns means getting less and less in return for increased effort. Twenty to thirty minutes of running three times per week should be enough to vascularize the heart and lungs 80 percent and achieve a resting pulse rate in the low sixties. Competitive athletes exceed this point to shave seconds off their racing times, but most people won't benefit much from such effort. Monitoring progress using the five tests suggested by this book is likely to show whether your cardio exertion is adequate. Adding an hour or more of weight training before or after cardio gives you a much better return on your effort than more cardio.

Section D:

Muscle-Fat Composition and Nutrition

CHAPTER 9

FATS IN YOUR DIET

Lipids include all fatlike chemical compounds that are insoluble in water, such as fats and oils that are primarily triglycerides, waxes of animal or plant origin, phospholipids, sterols (e.g., cholesterol), and fatty acids. Many different types of lipids, provided by the foods we eat or produced within the body, are absolutely necessary for our proper function.

The nature and function of lipids depends on molecular composition. Some are structured to carry and move fat-soluble vitamins (A, D, E, K) through the bloodstream to their target sites. Some function as antioxidants. Others are configured to be incorporated as structural components of the brain and body cell membranes, where they control inflammation and blood clotting and contribute to brain development and function.

Fats are a major source of fuel (energy) for the body's metabolic processes, because they provide *nine calories per gram*—more than twice what the same mass of carbohydrates or protein provides. Certain fats serve as storage for the body's extra calories until they are needed. Meanwhile, in this state, they fill fat cells (adipose tissue) that help insulate the body and cushion internal organs against physical trauma. Fats are responsible for many other important functions in the body. However, as necessary as they are, fats can also harm the body if consumed improperly. You must be just as judicious about the *type* of fat you consume as the *quantity*.

Dietary Cholesterol

Cholesterol, a fatty acid, is found in all body tissues, especially the liver, blood, and brain, where it helps to organize cell membranes and control their permeability, which is crucial to the body's survival. Cholesterol derivatives in the skin convert to vitamin D_3 when the skin is exposed to sunlight. Vitamin D_3 mediates intestinal calcium absorption and bone calcium metabolism.

Cholesterol also helps in the synthesis of essential compounds, such as bile acids and steroid hormones. Because cholesterol molecules are insoluble in blood, they attach themselves to protein molecules so that the blood can transport them where needed. The resultant composite molecule, soluble in blood, is called a *lipoprotein*. Different protein components can combine with cholesterol in different configurations to produce different types of lipoproteins with different properties. These are classified as either high density or low density, depending on their protein content. The more protein they have, the greater their density. Chapter 2 explained why we are especially interested in the lipoproteins LDL (Low Density Lipoprotein) and HDL (High Density Lipoprotein).

Where does the body obtain its cholesterol? Normally, the liver and other organs produce 80 percent of the body's cholesterol (which is a white, crystalline substance when isolated). Individual cells can also produce their own cholesterol. These sources produce enough to meet all the body's daily requirements, which might depend on a variety of factors such as weight training, for example, which raises the need for cholesterol because it leads to a significant replacement of millions of damaged cells (Chapters 11 and 12).

Another source is dietary cholesterol, which is present in animal foods, but not in plant foods. Foods with high levels of dietary cholesterol include egg yolks, organ meats, all animal fats, shellfish, squid, dairy products, and fatty meats. The body's production is *reduced by the amount consumed* in order to maintain inherent levels. However, if the amount of cholesterol consumed is greater than bodily needs, the excess will *increase* the blood's concentration of cholesterol. The same thing will occur if your body is genetically programmed to produce more than it needs. Higher concentrations of cholesterol in the blood significantly increase the risk of cardiovascular disease. Control cholesterol levels with a healthy diet lower in saturated and trans fats, higher in unsaturated fats, and exercise (Chapter 2). If your cholesterol—and thus LDL levels—cannot be controlled by diet and exercise, then medical intervention will be required.

Triglycerides

Triglycerides are not a type of cholesterol, but rather a type of fat also found in the blood. Your body makes some triglycerides, and some come from the food you eat. When you eat, your body uses some calories for immediate energy. If you take in more than it needs at a given time, it converts surplus calories into triglycerides and stores them *in fat cells* for later use. As a consequence, your blood triglyceride levels go up.

High triglyceride levels in the blood are associated with excess weight, excess alcohol consumption, high sugar consumption, and diabetes. If you have both high triglyceride and high LDL levels, your chances of having a heart attack increase. Triglycerides, at high levels, can be reduced by *30 percent to 40 percent* through exercise, largely through the loss of excess body fat. Your triglyceride level is usually measured at the same time as your blood cholesterol levels (i.e., HDL, LDL, and total), from the same blood sample.

Fat Composition

All fats are made up of a combination of saturated, monounsaturated, and polyunsaturated fatty acids, but one of the three usually predominates. The dominant type determines the physical characteristics of the fat. Fats containing a high proportion of saturated fatty acids, such as butter or lard, have a relatively high melting point and tend to be solid at room temperature. Most vegetable oils, which contain higher levels of monounsaturated or polyunsaturated fats, are usually liquid at room temperature.

Monounsaturated Fats

These types of fat have room for two additional hydrogen atoms per molecule. They have been shown to improve (*decrease*) blood cholesterol levels. They are found in olive oil, canola oil, peanut oil, nonhydrogenated margarine, avocados, and some nuts such as almonds, pistachios, pecans, and hazelnuts.

Polyunsaturated Fats

These types of fat have room for *more* than two additional hydrogen atoms per molecule. They can lower bad LDL cholesterol levels. One type of polyunsaturated fat is *omega-3*, which can help prevent the clotting of blood and help lower triglycerides. Sources of omega-3 are cold-water fish such as mackerel, sardines, herring, rainbow trout, and salmon, as well as canola and soybean oils, omega-3 eggs, flaxseed, walnuts, and pecans.

Another type of polyunsaturated fat is *omega-6*. It also helps lower LDL cholesterol, but in large amounts, it is also thought to lower supposed good HDL cholesterol. Eat omega-6 in moderation. It's found in safflower, sunflower, and corn oils; in nonhydrogenated margarine; and in almonds, pecans, Brazil nuts, and sunflower seeds.

Omega-3 and omega-6 are considered *essential* fatty acids because they cannot be made by the body and so must be provided by the diet.

Saturated Fat

The molecules of these fats have no room for extra hydrogen atoms, which is what "saturated" means. This category includes animal fats that have the consistency of butter at room temperature. They are important to the body; for example, some play an important role in supporting the immune system. Consumed in excessive amounts, however, they can *raise* the level of bad LDL cholesterol in the body. Foods high in saturated fat include fatty meats, full-fat dairy products, butter, hard margarines, lard, coconut oil, ghee (clarified butter), vegetable ghee, and palm oil.

Trans Fat

Trans fat and cis fat molecules, identical in their molecular composition, are mirror images of each other in three-dimensional space. Unsaturated fats are often hydrogenated (hydrogen atoms added to them) to prevent them from becoming rancid (to give them a longer shelf life). The problem is that the pressure, heat, and catalysts used in the hydrogenation process convert many normal, cis-structured fat molecules to abnormal, trans-structured fat molecules with *harmful biochemical properties*. Trans fats are therefore found in partially hydrogenated margarines, deep-fried foods from fast-food outlets (fries, doughnuts), and many packaged crackers, cookies, and commercially baked products.

Studies have shown that trans fats raise the level of "bad" LDL cholesterol, lower that of supposed "good" HDL, and increase triglyceride levels in the blood. Three strikes! Consequently, some scientists believe that trans fats create higher risk for coronary disease than excess saturated fats. Equally disturbing is that these abnormal trans-fat molecules displace the normal cis molecules required in cell membranes, a process that degrades the normal metabolic functions of the cell. For example, when they are incorporated into brain-cell membranes, they interfere with the ability of neurons to communicate with each other, causing neural degeneration and diminished mental performance and, potentially, neurodegenerative diseases such as multiple sclerosis, Alzheimer's disease, and Parkinson's disease. Trans fats are also suspected carcinogens.

Other Factors

Smoking, diabetes mellitus, alcohol, androgenic and anti-inflammatory steroids, excess weight, and emotional stress also have a negative influence on blood lipid levels. For women, menopause can worsen the blood lipid profile as estrogen levels decline.

Diet and Behavior Guidelines

The guidelines below aim to reduce your risk of cardiovascular disease. Although we still need more research on the role of fats in metabolism, in the meantime, doctors and dieticians continue to recommend a low-fat diet and a healthy lifestyle.

You should apply the quantities I suggest proportionally to your daily calorie intake. A general rule of thumb is to multiply your body weight (in pounds) by ten for the daily calories you need to *maintain current weight*. If you are overweight as evidenced by your waist size, use prudent judgment: consume fewer calories than are provided by this formula. Aim for a deficit of one pound per week.

- Check nutrition labels on food packages for calorie content and fat composition.

- Your total fat intake should be no higher than 20 to 35 percent of your required daily calories.

- Choose healthy polyunsaturated (up to 10 percent) and monounsaturated fats (up to 20 percent), found mainly in vegetable oils, nuts, and fish.

- Limit your intake of saturated fat, found mainly in red meat and high-fat dairy products, to no more than 7 percent of daily calories.

- Avoid trans fats in foods made with shortening or partially hydrogenated vegetable oil, hard margarines, fast foods, and many premade foods.

- Use lower-fat cooking methods such as baking, broiling, or steaming. Avoid fried food.

- See your doctor as soon as you can for a checkup that includes blood tests and an assessment of your cardiovascular risk level (based on age, sex, stress level, smoking, alcohol consumption, personal health record, activity level, ethnicity, and family medical history). The sooner you know your risk level, the sooner you can start looking after yourself.

- Use your national food guide to plan a healthier diet. Eat more vegetables, fruit, and whole grains while keeping in mind that quantity is important. Excessive consumption converts to unwanted fat. Make sure this includes ten to twenty-five grams of soluble fiber per day, such as found in oat bran, oatmeal, rice bran, barley, beans, peas, citrus fruits, and strawberries.

Following these guidelines will have a definite impact on your cardiovascular health, but adding what I advise in the rest of this book will have an even greater influence.

CHAPTER 10

MUSCLE VERSUS FAT

Note that diet alone, a cardiovascular training regimen alone, or a combination of them without weight training, causes you to lose *muscle* as well as fat. This has to be avoided!

A proper training program that includes cardiovascular training in concert with weight training should cause you to lose fat while you gain muscle. The average person should try to add a reasonable *five to fifteen* pounds (or more) of skeletal muscle to his or her frame. Five or six hours of training per week should do it. (Bodybuilders train for twenty or more hours per week because they want much larger gains in muscle mass.)

Why and How?

How do you measure your loss of fat and gain of muscle? Let's see.

Regardless of what you eat, if you consume more calories in a day than you burn, they get stored as fat in different locations on the body, including the waist. Meanwhile, challenging weights in your training program increase your strength and (desirably) your muscle mass.

Remember that muscle weighs more than fat! This means that your weight increases for one of three reasons: your fat content has gone up, your muscle mass has gone up, or some combination of the two. An increase in the body's fat content always leads to an increase in waist size whereas an increase in muscle mass has negligible impact on waist size. To keep track of these muscle-fat changes, measure your waist and weigh yourself every day.

Here are four possible muscle-fat composition scenarios:

- **Your weight goes up while your waist goes down.** You are losing fat while you are increasing your muscle mass. This is ideal!

- **Your weight remains the same while your waist goes down.** You are losing fat and gaining muscle. This is excellent!

- **Your weight goes up while your waist also goes up.** Your fat content is definitely increasing, while your muscle mass might or might not be. Avoid this. Get that waist down!

- **Your weight goes down while your waist stays the same.** An interesting scenario! This means that your body's fat content is not changing, so, in effect, you must be losing muscle tissue. This can mean you are working too hard (probably at aerobic endurance training) and burning muscle tissue for energy while at the same time eating enough to maintain your fat component. Your waist circumference *might or might not be* an acceptable size while this is happening (refer to waist-hip ratio below).

Understanding these four scenarios will help you interpret properly any other scenarios that you might also encounter.

Waist-Hip Ratio

How small should your waist be? When should you be satisfied with your waist size? To calculate your waist-hip ratio, measure your waist at its smallest point and your hips at their widest point. Then, divide your waist measurement by your hip measurement. Dr. Yusuf's team found that a waist-hip ratio greater than .85 for women and .90 for men is strongly linked to an increased risk of cardiovascular disease. Your waist should definitely be smaller than your hips.

Footnote

I mentioned earlier (Chapter 7) that BMI and skinfold techniques provide unreliable assessments of fat content. The same can be said of electronic impedance instruments that use the resistance of fat to the passage of a mild current to measure fat content. Again, daily waist-weight measurements more effectively monitor changes in both fat and muscle content. You can quickly perceive the changes you want: an excellent motivator. But don't cheat. Make sure the tape is snug, but not so tight that it cuts into the soft part of your waist. You benefit much more from an honest measurement.

CHAPTER 11

MORE TIPS ON NUTRITION

Here are a few nutrition-related topics well worth considering as you are following your program.

Visceral Fat and Hunger

Within your abdomen, visceral fat surrounds your internal organs. It is not simply a passive deposit of stored energy. It is the worst kind of fat, because it tends to release fatty acids into the bloodstream. These substances are associated with high levels of cardiovascular mortality in both men and women. (Other killer diseases, such as type 2 diabetes and cancer, are also associated with excess calories and obesity.)

To get rid of toxic visceral fat, you must reduce your waistline. However, it is extremely difficult to lose fat by simply exercising it off with cardio. A pound of fat contains about 3,500 calories; there are 70,000 calories in 20 pounds. A 165-pound person burns 250 calories by jogging for half an hour. It would take *seven* hours of jogging to lose a pound of fat—a tall order! Shedding 20 pounds, if need be, would be a monumental task.

Exercise helps the process of weight loss, but not as much as people assume. It is better not to accumulate body fat in the first place. Try to avoid excessive hunger, which causes you to overeat:

- Eat breakfast every morning shortly after you get up

- Snack lightly only

This means five or six meals *including snacks* per day. Do not exceed your total allotted calories for the day. You'll soon know if you've gone overboard: your waist measurement will go up in the next couple of mornings. Losing weight retards hunger pangs, because you now have *less body mass to nourish*. Thus, the more weight you lose, the easier it becomes to avoid overeating and control your weight.

University of Western Ontario professor Kaiping Yang discovered that the kind of fat cells found in the abdomen produce a hormone (neuropeptide Y or NPY) that stimulates appetite when produced in the brain. We used to believe that appetite originated only in the brain. Worse, this hormone compounds the problem by stimulating the production of the type of fat cells that produce it. This implies that the smaller your waist, the less of this hormone is released, and the less likely you are to be hungry. However, Dr. Yang reminds us that the study was done on rats, not humans—and that his team did not specifically test to see if NPY produced by fat cells would stimulate appetite. But, given that NPY produced by fat cells is identical to NPY produced by the brain, we can assume that it works similarly.

Proteins and Amino Acids

Weight training, especially heavy weight training, causes microscopic tears in *millions* of muscle cells during each workout, over and above regular wear and tear, which is why you need a diet rich in protein or amino acids. The extra protein should provide a more efficient repair of the strained muscle fibers, and the production of new ones, to improve your strength. (However, avoid bodybuilder consumption guidelines for proteins or amino acids. They work out twenty or more hours per week, compared with your six or so.) The membranes of these new cells require cholesterol (Chapter 9). Weight training consistently for long periods might therefore help reduce cholesterol levels.

Resting Metabolic Rate

"Metabolism" is the sum of all the biochemical reactions in your body that maintain life. These reactions require energy to burn calories, and hence fat, but at a variable rate. The more active you are, the higher the rate. Your resting metabolic rate (RMR) is the lowest, but it accounts for about 70 percent of your total daily metabolism, so it is a major factor in controlling your level of body fat. The more you raise your RMR, the more fat you burn, both at rest and while active.

You can raise RMR in a variety of ways:

- Weight train with intensity. After that, your RMR remains higher for two days or more. A cardio workout does not have the same effect.

- Add muscle tissue. A pound of muscle burns, on average, about ten times more calories per day than a pound of fat.

- Eat breakfast. It boosts your metabolic rate by about 5 percent.

- Eat protein. It has been estimated that thirty calories are required to digest and assimilate a hundred calories of protein, but only six are needed per hundred calories of carbohydrates. Include protein in each meal and snack.

- Drink water. Properly diluted blood and other body fluids make your biochemical processes more efficient. Drink water regularly while you are working out.

Your RMR slows down as you get older, by 0.5 percent or more a year, making it more difficult for you to control your body weight. Proper exercise that maintains muscle mass can help maintain your RMR over time, though.

Footnote

It is fine and dandy for me to recommend the above guidelines, but in the final analysis, your own self-discipline will be the deciding factor. That cannot be avoided!

Section E:
Weight-Training Principles

CHAPTER 12

BASIC WEIGHT-TRAINING PRINCIPLES AND DEFINITIONS

This chapter provides a short fitness lexicon explaining important concepts mentioned in earlier chapters and employed in the chapters that follow.

Muscle Strength is a measure of the force a muscle, or group of muscles, is capable of exerting against a resistance through the leverage of one or more skeletal joints. This force can vary from slightly more than the resistance to a maximum force depending on how fast the individual wants to move the resistance. In an isometric contraction the force is less or equal to the resistance it is opposing which is why movement does not occur.

Muscular Endurance refers to the number of times a muscle can contract consecutively, without rest, before it is forced to stop *involuntarily* (due to muscular exhaustion) by an excessive build-up of lactic acid. The more often it can contract for a given resistance, the more muscular endurance it is said to have. Both improved vascularization and improved strength increase muscular endurance.

All-out sprinting is an activity requiring good muscular endurance as opposed to cardiovascular endurance—which is a measure of your capacity to maintain a long-term, low-intensity activity (such as jogging).

The Overload Principle is making a muscle contract with a force greater than that needed to simply move its usual limb weight. Imagine you are standing upright, with your right arm hanging straight down. To flex it ninety degrees or more, the biceps muscle normally contracts with at least enough force to pull your right forearm (which weighs about five pounds) upward. Now, do it again, but holding a five-pound dumbbell. The biceps now has to contract with a force at least slightly greater than ten pounds to lift both the right forearm and the weight. The faster you want to lift the weight, the more of the biceps muscle your brain must solicit: you have overloaded your right biceps.

The dumbbell is a form of *resistance* (i.e., to movement). Used in properly designed exercises, resistance can overload—and strengthen—any of the body's skeletal muscles. Any number of things—cast iron plates, rubber bands, weighted belts, your own body weight, etc.—can serve as resistance against a movement initiated by the contraction of one muscle or a combination of them. Thanks to Mother Nature, the greater the resistance used over time, the larger and stronger any worked muscle becomes—hypertrophy ("bulk up"). On the other hand if, after having overloaded and hypertrophied a muscle for a period of time, you need to reduce the resistance possibly because of an injury, the muscle will get smaller—atrophy—in line with the drop in resistance.

The Progressive Overload Principle is the process of gradually increasing resistance, over weeks and months, to obtain a corresponding increase in the strength, bulk, and muscular endurance of a muscle. For example, once you can do ten or more consecutive reps of an exercise to failure, you are almost ready to increase the resistance (*do not rush it!*). Continue to use the original weight for at least three more sessions before you increase the weight. The target number of repetitions is based on your objectives (see Chapters 15, 16, and 17).

The heavier weight should feel *no tougher* to lift, mentally or physically, than the previous weight, as long as you increase the resistance in small increments. Note, however, as you might expect, that the number of reps you can do for the same exercise with the increased weight will probably fall to seven or eight. Keep working until you're back up to ten, and then increase the resistance again. This may take a couple of weeks. Otherwise if you always work out with the same weight (no progression), your strength and level of vascularization will barely improve over time.

In response to the Progressive Overload Principle, *larger* muscles bulk up more, and hence add more muscle mass to the body than smaller ones. For example, thighs (quadriceps) bulk up much more than calves when you work them with equal intensity (not with the same weight: quadriceps are inherently much stronger than calf muscles). Thus, working the largest muscles gives a greater vascularized muscle mass, and hence a greater reduction in blood pressure. When you start a program, you need about two months of progressive overloading before you get to weights that are heavy enough to bulk you up and significantly vascularize your muscles. As mentioned in the preface, resistance training does not bulk up women because their hormone balance is different from men's.

An aside: If you intend a career in health, fitness, or sports, I strongly recommend that you lift weights for at least one year using the progressive overload system to really understand the impact of a good weight-training program on the body and the associated physiology. It is much better to speak from experience when teaching these principles to others.

CAUTION

Be careful with a new, heavier weight when you progressively overload a muscle! The initial stages of using higher weight are when you are at greatest risk of injury, especially if the increase is too large. The muscles and their tendons have not yet adapted to the new and more challenging resistance. Do not go to *failure* with the new weight until after a couple of sessions.

Lifting to Failure

Lifting to failure is the real key to improving strength and vascularizing muscles more efficiently. "Failure" is when you cannot do another repetition at the end of a set because of fatigue. As we've seen, lactic acid buildup is the cause; this is what stimulates muscle development. Maximum intensity for a set involves going to failure with the weight.

To stress muscles to their limit and get even better results, a lifter might ask a spotter (helper) to assist with an additional two or three reps of a particular set after the failure point. The spotter should use the fingers to lift just enough on the resistance to keep it moving while the lifter does most of the pushing. This is done only when it is obvious the lifter has reached failure. As long as a lifter can complete a rep without help, he or she should do so; the workout will be much more effective.

Specificity

A muscle can be trained to contract more forcefully in a specific direction. The direction desired depends on the lifter's objectives. For example, in track and field, the shot put is best thrown at forty-five degrees to the horizontal for maximum distance. Thus the shot-putter should train the pectoral and triceps muscles on a bench sloped to provide that angle of push (bench press, Chapters 13 and 17).

Isometric versus Isotonic Training

Isometric training involves contracting muscles as completely as possible against an immovable resistance for ten to fifteen seconds. Although this is probably the best way to improve strength, its disadvantage is that it has too *much* specificity: it enhances a muscle's strength in one direction only. To improve performance in a physical skill that requires strength through a particular muscle's full or partial range of movement, an isometric exercise would have to be done at six or more different positions. This is time-consuming.

The second and most realistic approach is isotonic training, in which the contracting muscle actually moves the resistance through its full (or partial) range of movement, as in traditional weight training.

However, the isometric principle can be taken advantage of: when a weight has been lifted to failure isotonically, the lifter can continue to push against the static weight for ten seconds or so before returning it to its starting position—another way to enhance strength and vascularization!

Range of Motion

I recommend that you use a full range of movement for an exercise whenever possible. It trains the whole muscle rather than just a part of it. For example, in flies on the Pec Dec machine (illustrated in Chapter 17), most people move both arms inward at the same time and stop the movement when the grips meet in front of the face. Instead, you should alternate the arms one at a time, and each time, continue the full movement *to the opposite shoulder*. To get a feel for this suggestion, place your hand on the pectoral muscle as you are moving the grip with the opposite hand through the recommended full range of movement. You will feel the sequence of contraction of different parts of the pectoral muscle as the flies movement progresses from start to finish. Working the whole muscle rather than just half vascularizes a larger mass.

Breathing

Never hold your breath while you are weight training. Strenuous effort of this type requires that you breathe well during the exercise to provide necessary oxygen (Chapter 3) to the mitochondrion of the working muscles. Thus, for each repetition, exhale as you lift the weight and inhale as you return it to its initial position.

Pyramid Down

Assume you are doing three sets of an exercise. Pyramiding down means that you reduce the weight you use for the next consecutive set of the same exercise, during that same training session. The amount by which you pyramid down depends on the exercise. The new weight should allow you to do *as many reps* as you did in the preceding set. Trial and error over weeks of weight training will allow you to better judge the amount required. It is an effective way to build strength and vascularize muscle. This technique is included for some exercises in the program found in Chapter 17.

Recovery

In the early stages of your program, expect to awaken feeling stiff and sore the day after a workout. This is caused largely by the fact that millions of muscle cells are torn during each session. They require a day or so to repair themselves. This is normal and might last more than a month, but keep it to a minimum by starting your program with *light weights* and progressing slowly.

For proper recovery, give a worked muscle at least one day's rest between workouts.

For proper physical and mental recuperation, take a week off every six or more weeks. Your progress in ensuing sessions should actually improve, because muscle tissue recuperates and bulks up more fully during this extended rest period. As a matter of fact two weeks now and again would not hurt.

Adhesions

Adjacent parallel muscle cells are designed to slide easily over each other as the muscle contracts or relaxes. However, while healing, some adjacent cells may actually fuse together. As you might expect, the next time a muscle with such adhesions is called into action, the stress will actually tear many of these apart. Post-exercise (or post-physical work) soreness and stiffness that occurs for a couple of days afterwards is therefore not just caused by damaged cells but also by the tearing of these adhesions.

Overtraining

Overtraining is more likely if you work out excessively without taking necessary breaks. As previously mentioned each weight-training session damages millions of muscle cells. If they are not given the time to repair themselves, the damage can accumulate. Quite severe symptoms can result, including chronic fatigue, insomnia, loss of appetite, and proneness to injury. Muscles ache, body weight and strength drop, and you tend to lose interest in your training. Your resting blood pressure and resting pulse rate may also increase chronically, but only until you no longer feel the overtraining symptoms.

If you experience these symptoms, you should definitely take at least one (preferably two or more) weeks off. When you return to your program, reduce your workload by decreasing the number of workouts, the number of exercises, the number of sets, and/or the resistance you are using. Experiment, but take the required rest periods!

Multimuscle Exercises

Actions initiated by muscles are either of the single-muscle or multiple-muscle variety. Strict biceps curls are a good example of single-muscle action, as the biceps are the only prime movers that contract during the exercise (Chapter 14).

On the other hand, multimuscle exercises require a coordinated effort on the part of two or more muscles. Either a group of muscles works *concurrently* to lift a weight, or the muscles contract *consecutively* (in series, one after the other, from start to finish) to eventually complete a lift. An example of muscles working concurrently is the bench press, where the front deltoids, pectorals, and triceps work in almost perfect unison to lift the bar. Of the exercises in my program, upright rowing is a good example of muscles working consecutively, or in series. Although there is some overlap, the biceps start the lift, followed by the medial deltoids. The upper trapezius then takes over to complete the lift.

Detraining

A return to a sedentary lifestyle means the body will gradually return to its original unfit state. That is, muscles will atrophy (get smaller) and become weaker; vascularization and functionality will also decline accordingly. Systolic pressure and diastolic blood pressure will rise.

CHAPTER 13

TRAINING THE WHOLE MUSCLE

To reduce blood pressure effectively, it is important to train and vascularize as much muscle mass as possible. This chapter explains how to design your program to train a complete muscle by choosing exercises according to the *alignment* of its cells. More than one exercise may be needed for this. First some basic information!

Motor Units

A motor unit is a group of muscle fibers that can be made to contract simultaneously by *one* single nerve cell. Individual skeletal muscles are composed of many motor units. For finely skilled movements, the motor units are composed of only a few muscle fibers per nerve (for example, movements controlled by the extrinsic muscles of the eye). The muscles used for gross motor skills, such as kicking a ball, might be made up of motor units composed of as many as eight hundred or more muscle fibers *per nerve*. This provides more strength, but at the expense of precision of movement.

Motor units also control the force of a skeletal muscle's contraction. The heavier the weight you lift or the faster you want to lift it, the more motor units the central nervous system calls into play. A feedback system tells the brain if more effort is needed as the attempt progresses..

Muscle Fiber Alignment

Understanding the principle of muscle fiber alignment is essential to the design of an effective weight-training program. No doubt you've seen many anatomical diagrams of skeletal muscles that also clearly illustrate their *striations*. See below the diagram of the left and right sides of the pectoralis major (chest) muscle. Each striation is a bundle of parallel muscle fibers (cells), each as long as the muscle. As you can see, the pectoral's striations, and hence its muscle fibers, line up in a variety of directions.

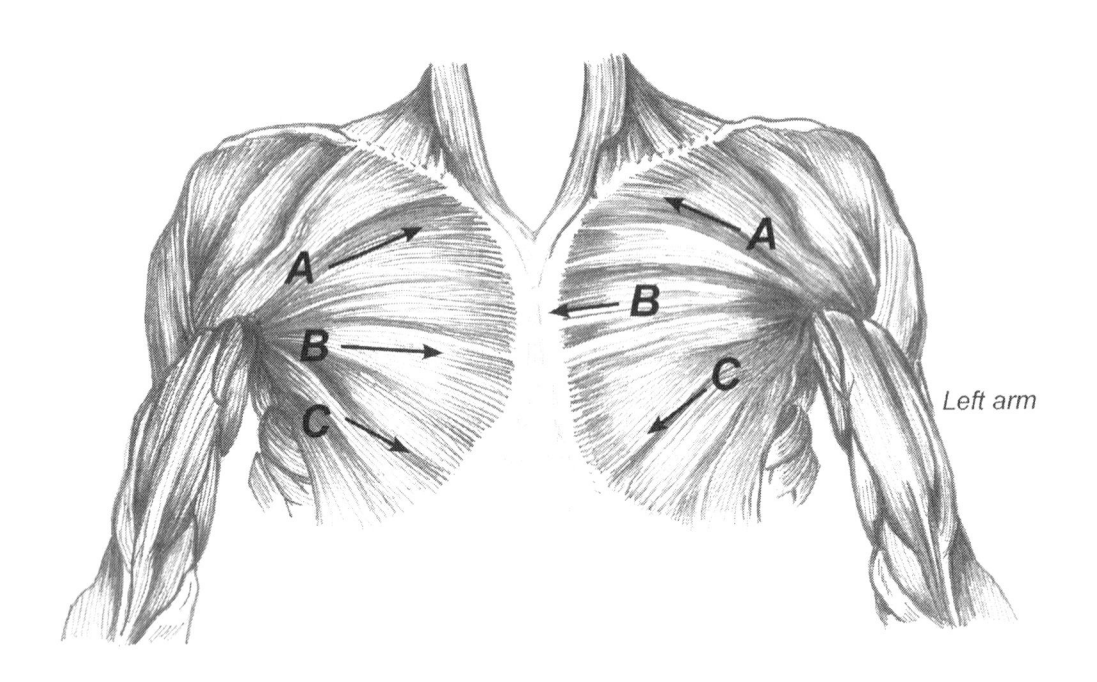

Left arm

Generally speaking, each of the striations or bundles is attached to the skeleton at either end. One end (the *origin*) is fixed; the other (the *insertion*) is mobile.

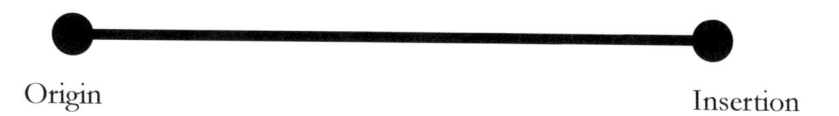

Origin   Insertion

When the muscle fibers of a striation are stimulated into action by a nerve impulse, they contract completely into a shorter, "fatter" shape. This forcefully pulls the insertion toward the origin, as illustrated by the arrow in the following sketch. This is how skeletal muscles create movement.

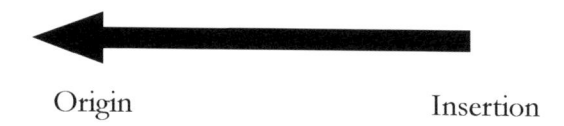

Origin   Insertion

In the diagram of the pectoral muscles, the striations of the left pectoral muscle that controls left-arm movements are divided conveniently into three broad areas: A, B, and C (upper, middle, and lower pecs). The origins of each of these striations are attached to the sternum or clavicle in the center region of the chest. The arrows extending from the letters found on the left pectoral indicate the direction of pull on the left arm when the fibers in a particular area contract to pull their insertions toward their origins. The same argument can be made for the right arm.

Using the example of the pectoral muscle, I explain below how its divisions control certain arm movements for the bench press performed at three different angles (scenarios 1 to 3).

Scenario 1: Regular Bench Press

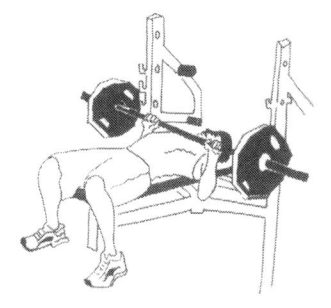

Starting position   **Direction and range of press**

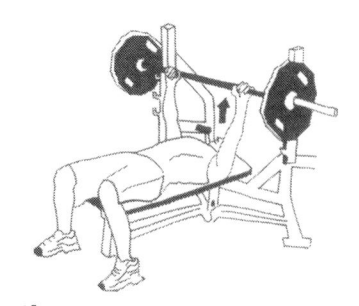

The first diagram shows a lifter in the starting position on a horizontal bench, ready to perform the regular bench press exercise. To attain this position, while holding the bar with a slightly greater-than-shoulder-width grip, the lifter has lowered the weight until the bar just touches the highest point of his chest. In this position, his upper arms are at forty-five degrees to the sides of his torso, as shown. From here, the lifting action involves pulling both upper arms backward and up while the triceps extend the complete arm to a vertical position.

To accomplish this, the lifter's brain must recruit the pectoral muscle cells that are best aligned, and hence best suited, for this purpose. The previous striated chest diagram shows us that regions A are best suited to pull the upper arms backward when they contract while the region B muscle cells pull them upward and inward. Because they experience the greatest resistance due to gravity during this movement, the bulk of the force must be supplied by the muscle cells of region B. Region C's contribution is negligible. Hence, to hypertrophy, strengthen, and vascularize the prime movers (Chapter 14) for this action, regions A (upper pecs) and especially B (middle pecs) on both sides, this is the action a lifter should *overload* (Chapter 12).

Scenario 2: Decline Bench Press

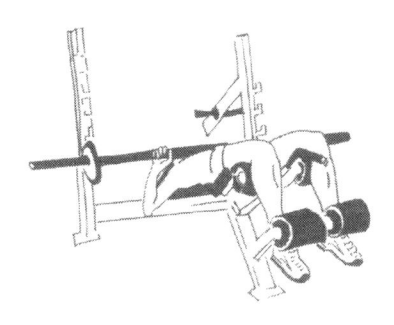

Starting position

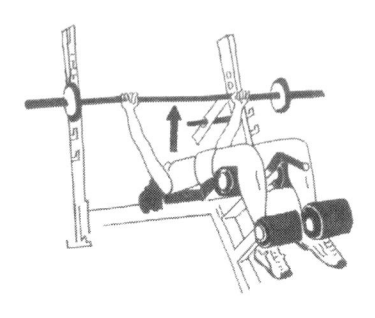

Direction and range of press

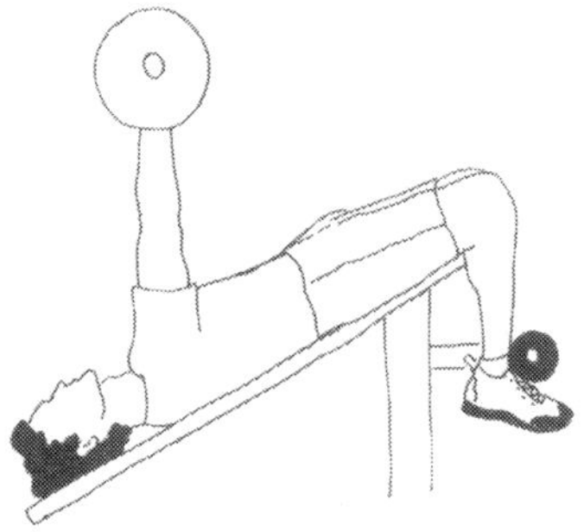

Side view

On a "decline bench" set at about a thirty-degree tilt, the lifter's head is lower than his knees while he uses the same lower position and arm action as in the regular bench press. However, the decline position requires different muscle cell recruitment by the brain: region C along with the lower part of region B pull the upper arms backward and upward, while the triceps extend the complete arm vertically upward. Thus, region C muscle cells experience the greatest resistance due to gravity and do the bulk of the lifting (see the simplified side-view diagram shown above). To hypertrophy, strengthen and vascularize region C (lower pecs) and to a lesser extent the lower part of region B (middle pecs), this movement is the one you *overload*.

Scenario 3: Incline Bench Press

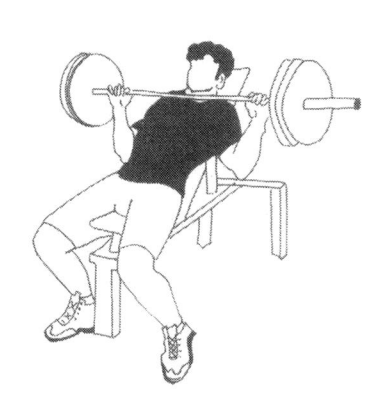

Starting position 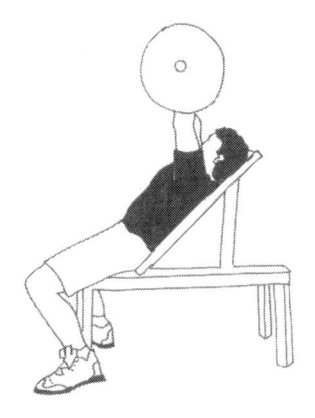   **Side view**

Conversely, for the incline bench press, the head is higher than the knees. This alignment means that for the lift, the brain's recruitment of muscle cells here emphasizes region A, as it is best suited for pulling the upper arms backward and upward, while the triceps extend the arm to a vertical position (the upper part of region B assists). Because region A encounters the most resistance due to gravity, it does the bulk of the lifting. Hence, to hypertrophy, strengthen, and vascularize especially region A (upper pecs) and the upper part of region B (middle pecs), this is the movement you *overload*.

A Multimuscle Perspective

Fibers of different muscles, although lined up in different directions, can also work together to create movement in a *single* direction. For example, different parts of the trapezius, rhomboid, latissimus dorsi, and posterior deltoid muscles of the upper back need to contract together to execute reverse flies (that is, to pull the upper arms upward and back toward the midline of the back while the upper body is inclined forward). The triceps extend the arms as they move upward. This exercise will tend to hypertrophy, strengthen, and vascularize the parts of these muscles that are used in the lift.

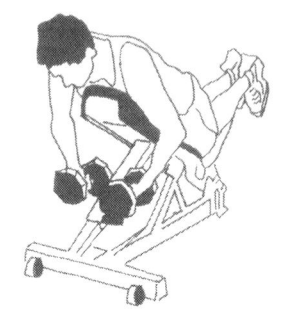

Starting position   **Direction and range of the side lifts**

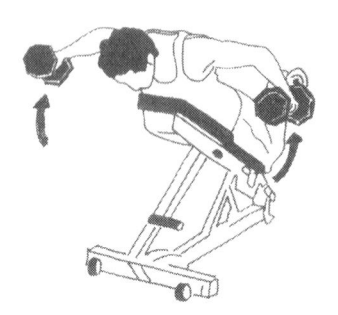

Back muscles

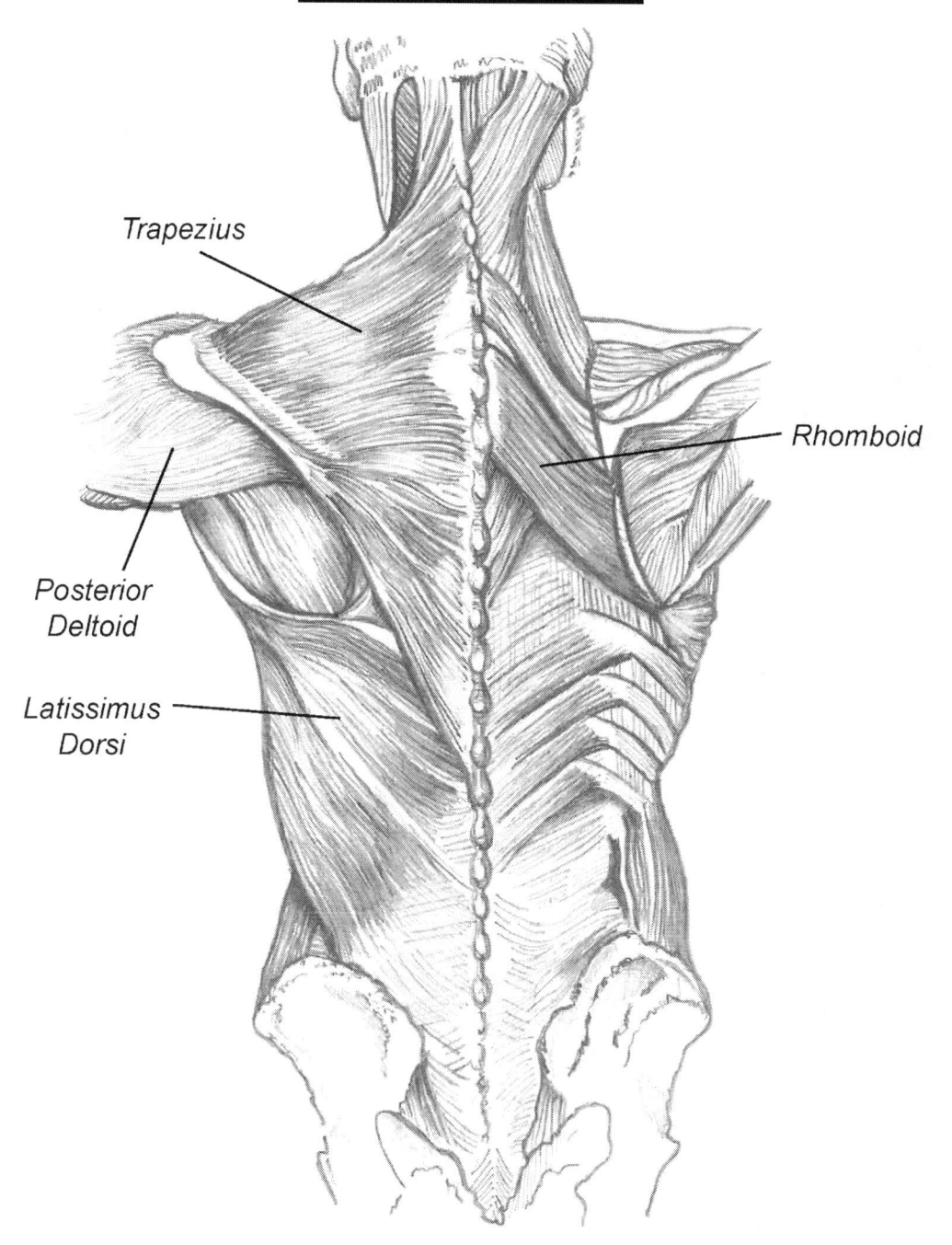

Trapezius

Rhomboid

Posterior Deltoid

Latissimus Dorsi

As you might suspect, these muscles can work together in a variety of combinations and create movement in many different directions.

85

CHAPTER 14

DIMENSIONS OF MUSCLE-INITIATED MOVEMENT

We've considered skeletal muscle movement at the motor unit level; we now examine it at a higher, more comprehensive level that is also essential to the design of an effective weight-training program.

Prime Movers and Stabilizers

In every movement initiated by the skeletal muscles, one or more muscles are *prime movers* and others are *stabilizers*. The prime movers execute the desired movement, whereas the stabilizers anchor the body, or parts of the body, to allow the desired movement to occur. For example, the weights used in strict biceps curls in the standing position would probably pull the lifter forward (to fall flat on his or her chest) were it not for stabilizer muscles that pull in the opposite direction, contracting partially to keep the body erect. These are the upper and lower back and posterior and anterior deltoid muscles, as well as the gluteal and hamstring muscles. The abdominals and pectorals also play a role. As you might suspect, the biceps muscles are the prime movers during this exercise. In all weight-training exercises, stabilizers benefit slightly from the exercise, but *not nearly as much* as the prime movers that the exercise targets much more directly.

Agonists and Antagonists

Muscles essentially work in pairs to perform their tasks. The *agonist* is responsible for the desired motion (the prime mover), while the *antagonist* acts against the agonist for fine control and balance. Such pairs can also be referred to as "opposing muscles." For example, when the biceps contracts to flex (bend) the arm, the triceps at the back of the same arm either relaxes completely to give the biceps full freedom of movement, *or* contracts enough to control the biceps' rate of *flexion*. Here, the biceps is considered the agonist and the triceps its antagonist. However, in the arm *extension*, the triceps is the agonist, and the biceps it is paired with is now the antagonist: their roles have been reversed. Another well-known agonist-antagonist pair is the pectorals of the chest versus the upper back muscles.

Muscle Tone

Muscle tone is the readiness of a muscle to contract. Even when a muscle is not being used, a small number of its motor units are always involuntarily activated to produce a sustained contraction of its fibers. While the muscle is at rest, it maintains tone with small groups of motor units that are *alternately* active and inactive in a constantly shifting pattern. Although the tension is not strong enough to produce movement, the muscle is always prepared for contraction, allowing for a quicker response. Muscle tone increases chronically with strength training.

Postural Considerations

The stronger a muscle becomes, the *chronically* shorter it remains while at rest, due to enhanced muscle tone. More of its motor units are activated while it is at rest. Understanding this is crucial for your posture. For example, if you only worked the pectorals and never their antagonists (the large upper back muscles), they would shorten chronically at rest, and you would create an imbalance; your shoulders would *hunch in* chronically toward your sternum. You would walk around this way.

To avoid imbalance between agonist and antagonist to maintain proper posture, you must work the antagonist as well as the agonist—in this example, the rhomboid, trapezius, posterior deltoid, and, to a certain extent, the latissimus dorsi. The same is true of all agonist-antagonist combinations.

Concentric, Eccentric, and Isometric Contraction

A muscle contraction is *concentric* when it shortens to apply its force (as for a biceps curl); this is our traditional perception of muscle action. An *eccentric* contraction is when a muscle's length increases while applying a force. For example, from the top of a just-completed biceps curl, the biceps contracts as it lengthens to control the weight's speed of descent as it is slowly lowered back to its original starting position. This is protection against a free drop that would no doubt injure the biceps muscle. This action is also called a *"negative rep"* and is great for strengthening the tendons. When climbing stairs, the quadriceps of the upper leg contract concentrically to lift one's body weight upwards for each stair; when going down stairs, the same quadriceps contract eccentrically to control descent and thereby prevent the individual from falling down the stairs. Specificity (Chapter 12) would suggest that different exercises overloading each action separately would be required to strengthen these different movements.

In an *isometric* contraction, the muscle does not change its length: movement does not take place (for example, while you push against an immovable object, such as a wall).

Section F:

Fitness Programs

PART 1: TYPES OF FITNESS PROGRAMS

CHAPTER 15

CHOOSING A FITNESS PROGRAM FOR A SPECIFIC SPORT

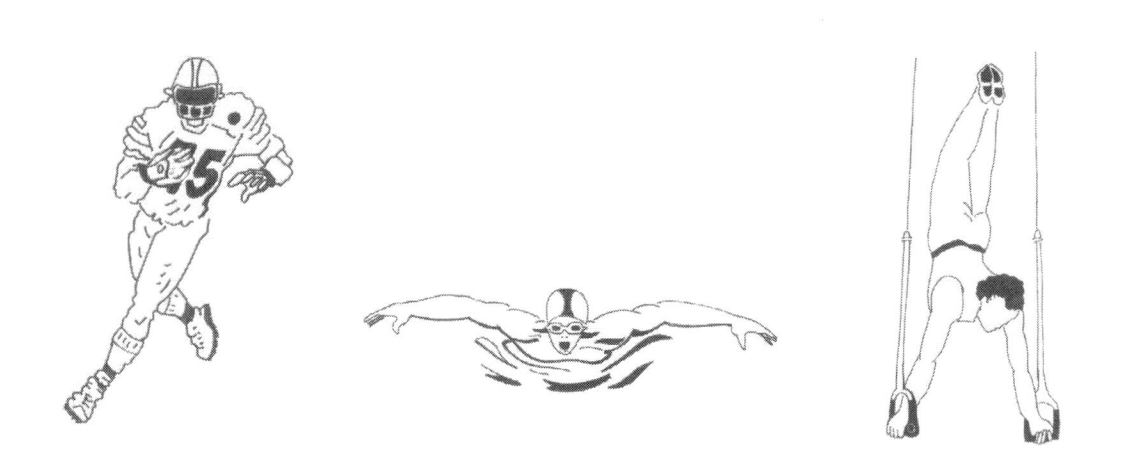

When you design a fitness program, your objectives are important. Do you want to improve your performance in a particular sport, or protect your health and improve your quality of life? A fitness program must be designed properly to achieve the desired results.

If you're seeking improved performance in a sport, you must first analyze the sport's general performance requirements. Below, I offer some brief examples to help you understand that different objectives call for differently designed programs.

For example, a *gymnast* wants to become as strong as possible without increasing body weight; he or she needs to maneuver the body with ease. Thus, weight training will involve sets of many repetitions with lighter weights to avoid bulking up too much. The body should be light as well as strong. Although muscle tone is very important in gymnastics, so is cardiovascular endurance. Fatigue, especially toward the end of a gymnastics routine, breeds errors.

A *professional wrestler* needs strength with minimum body fat. To be stronger and more agile than an opponent, wrestlers should use heavy weights with few repetitions per set and gain as little fat as possible. Cardiovascular fitness is very important to protect against fatigue as a match progresses. The less tired a wrestler is, the sharper he is during a bout.

If a *marathon runner* weight trains, the program should be similar to the gymnast's. Muscle tone is important, especially in the legs, but the body should be light as it must be carried a long distance. Diet should be low in fat and overall quantity. Cardiovascular fitness is paramount here.

For a *football lineman*, strength and body weight are both important. Much like a professional wrestler, he should weight train using few repetitions and heavy weights to gain strength and bulk. Body fat should be low for maximum agility. Cardiovascular fitness, although important for health, is only moderately important for a lineman's position, since he gets to rest often between plays.

A *quarterback* needs to be strong, but much more agile than his teammates on the line. To avoid bulking up too much, he should use moderately heavy weights in his workout, leaning toward ten reps or so per set (as opposed to six for a lineman). Cardiovascular fitness is very important to a quarterback's performance, as fatigue breeds errors, especially late in the game.

A *bodybuilder* targets specific muscles in very specific directions to make them as visible as possible during stage presentations. Posing successfully is the number one priority. The body has more than six hundred muscles, and a bodybuilder would train them all as specifically as possible if there were time (there isn't!). Obviously, body fat is kept to the very minimum for proper muscle definition—the striations are visible. Cardiovascular endurance is moderately important for success here, because it allows a bodybuilder to train for long periods.

For any sport, its skills determine which specific exercises the athlete should use in a fitness program. Using specificity, weight-training exercises should duplicate the sport's skills as closely as possible: overloading should cause the muscles to apply a force in the same direction they are applied in the skill. (Beyond the fitness program, the athlete must, of course, practice the actual sport in game-like conditions.)

CHAPTER 16

CHOOSING A FITNESS PROGRAM FOR HEALTH AND QUALITY OF LIFE

For your health and quality of life, your fitness program should aim to improve the following:

- cardiovascular endurance and energy level
- strength and muscular endurance
- body fat percentage
- bone density
- posture
- agility
- balance and flexibility
- level of concentration
- hand-eye coordination
- discipline, perseverance, and tenacity

Developing these qualities should make you a more active, functional, lucid, and self-reliant person with better self-esteem, for years to come. *Functionality* is the capacity to carry out daily, regular, job-related activities or recreational activities. Improvements in these areas should also reduce your risk of injury (for the older and frail, this includes the ability, for example, to avoid falls that might lead to bone fractures) during physical activity and protect you against a variety of illnesses, especially cardiovascular disease.

Here are some guidelines for developing a good fitness program:

Warm-Up and Flexibility

The warm-up should raise your body temperature to the point of mild perspiration without tiring you. (You may want to ask a physiotherapist to recommend exercises that help stabilize the lower back.)

As with any sport, reduce the possibility of injury during your workout by stretching many of the muscles and tendons you're about to train: this improves their *elasticity*, making them less susceptible to tears during stress. You should stretch a muscle for thirty seconds (count "one thousand one" to "one thousand thirty" to yourself as you stretch). Also, pay attention to your muscle's stretch reflex. A muscle can contract involuntarily while it is being pulled or stretched, which may strain it significantly. Stretch slowly, but never to the point of pain. *Do not bounce!*

You might find that you can stretch one side of the body more than the other (this can be the result of uneven daily habits, such as always carrying objects with your right hand). This structural imbalance can cause distortions (protrusion, herniation, rupture) in one or more lumbar discs while exercising, putting pressure on spinal nerves and/or the spinal cord that might lead to lower back pain. To correct this, stretch your least flexible side longer so that over time it will become as flexible as the other side. Take the time to analyze your daily activities to see if you need to modify them.

You must stretch at least three times per week for months to achieve long-term lengthening of muscles, tendons, or ligaments. For this reason, I stick with the same stretching exercises over time.

Crunches are a good warm-up exercise. They are like sit-ups, but done without hooking your feet under a support. To ensure that you actually work the abdominals and not the iliopsoas and associated muscles (hip flexors), do crunches with your feet on top of a bench. These are excellent for your lower back because they chronically shorten the abdominal muscles through increased muscle tone and pull your pelvic girdle into proper postural position while you are standing to lessen the strain on your lower back. Conversely, weak abs and a large stomach tend to increase the forward tilt of the pelvic girdle, making you very susceptible to back injury. Separate exercises are available to work the hip flexors (iliopsas) if need be.

Strength and Muscular Endurance

Resistance training (which usually means with weights) improves strength and muscular endurance: you burn more calories during workouts, resting metabolism of muscle tissue improves to help control body fat, and functionality improves. The heavier the weights you lift, the more the stressed muscles strengthen and bulk up to further enhance these benefits; again, I recommend that you increase your muscle mass by *five to fifteen pounds* (or more).

An aside: A 2011 study from the University of California published in the *Journal of Clinical Endocrinology & Metabolism* found that the greater an individual's total muscle mass, the lower the person's risk of insulin resistance, the major precursor of type 2 diabetes.

Important: Low blood pressure values resulting from vascularization in response to proper cardio and weight-training programs are a desired objective regardless of how low they drop. *The lower the better!* On the other hand, low blood pressure values that cause weakness or dizziness are related to illness and need a doctor's attention.

A good weight-training program aimed at developing strength, bulk, and muscular endurance in the large muscle groups can also easily offset the degenerative loss of muscle mass and strength that comes with age (*sarcopenia*). Beginning insidiously in one's forties and fifties, both men and women lose about 12 percent of their strength every ten years. Maintain your performance level and cardiovascular health by conserving muscle mass.

Heavier weights, among other things, also promote enhanced metabolism of calcium and the development of good, strong, dense bones to help prevent osteoporosis. A weight you can work for at least ten reps per exercise should be adequate. You should understand, though, that the term "heavy weight" is relative. What is heavy for one person might be light for another. Each will benefit equally well, as long as each lifter reaches failure during a set.

Exercises should work the parts of the body in a balanced fashion: the chest and its antagonist, the back; the shoulders (front, back, and side deltoids); the quadriceps (upper front of the leg) and their antagonists, the hamstrings (upper back of the leg); the biceps (upper front of the arm) and their antagonists, the triceps (upper back of the arm). The calves already get sufficient work from walking or jogging in the cardiovascular phase, and the forearms are worked enough simply by gripping the bar during lifting, so you don't need to add exercises for them.

Your goal should be to progressively increase your strength and muscular endurance by increasing the weight you lift, as explained in Chapter 12. Remember not to increase by too much!

Cardiovascular Fitness

As explained in earlier chapters both endurance and resistance (ex. weight training) activities contribute to your cardiovascular fitness. They should be *intense* enough to reduce your resting pulse rate and resting blood pressure gradually over the weeks (Chapters 2 & 7). A 2006 University of Illinois study showed that cardiovascular activity actually adds new functional neurons to the brain, increasing a person's memory and cognitive ability—so it has even more benefits than just vascularizing your heart and lungs.

Note that activities that burn exactly the same number of calories do not necessarily have identical impacts on the body. Walking a mile briskly burns almost the same number of calories as if you run the same distance at a demanding pace. However, the demanding run has the added advantage of vascularizing the heart and lungs, which is much more beneficial for the cardiovascular system (and it tones some skeletal muscles).

Concentration and Hand-Eye Coordination

One great way to enhance concentration and hand-eye coordination is to use a punching speed bag for eight minutes or so at the end of your regular workout, while you are tired. This forces the taxed brain to concentrate for that period. In the long run, this could help alleviate possible degenerative neurological problems. (Beats doing crossword puzzles!) It is also fun and a good conditioning activity for the shoulders. You can become fairly adept at this skill even with a minimum of instruction. Just start slowly. (A short workout of simple martial arts skills or skipping rope would provide the same benefits.)

Agility

I also recommend that you work on improving your agility. You might try adapting your new capabilities (strength, cardiovascular endurance, muscular endurance, flexibility, concentration, etc.) to an activity that requires them. You could do, say, ten minutes of simple gymnastics at the end of your workout, play tennis or soccer, or swim, dive, go hiking, and so on. Practical chores, such as mowing the lawn, shovelling snow, chopping wood, etc., are also beneficial. Improved functionality is the objective.

Discipline, Perseverance, and Tenacity

A faithful, dedicated adherence to your fitness program will certainly enhance these attributes, adding significantly to your quality of life. Older people often avoid physical activities or skills they could do when they were young. We say that we are "too old to do this anymore." An attitude of reticence sets in. But if we boldly take on some of these challenges, we might surprise ourselves. Our self-esteem and functionality would improve.

For example, with perseverance, a former gymnast, myself, was able to do handstand push-ups against the wall almost as well as he used to. For other people, simpler gymnastics moves (e.g., front, back, or side rolls; cartwheels; headstands; hip circles on a high bar) that they used to do in physical education class might be the answer. Most sports have skills that could serve this purpose. If time allows, they could be an important component of a fitness workout.

Cool-Down

Muscles that have been worked with intensity swell slightly with blood for a half hour or more after the end of a workout. Weight lifters say they are "pumped up." This is the body's attempt to rid muscles of accumulated metabolites, such as lactic acid. However, it also hampers your circulation for that thirty minutes and tends to raise your blood pressure somewhat. Mild activities such as simple calisthenics or walking slowly on a treadmill for fifteen or twenty minutes will return your circulation to normal faster than if you do nothing. A warm shower also helps.

Note: Your pursuit of mobility, concentration, hand-eye coordination, perseverance, and tenacity should not distract you from the endurance and weight-training components of your fitness program. The latter are the most important to your cardiovascular health. If your time is limited, endurance and weight training should be your number-one priority.

According to Newton, a body at rest tends to stay at rest, whereas a body in motion tends to stay in motion. Do yourself a favor and get your body in motion.

PART 2: PERSONAL FITNESS PROGRAM

CHAPTER 17

MY PERSONAL FITNESS PROGRAM

A competitive bodybuilder trains three or more hours per day, five or six days a week, trying to work as many different muscles as possible. For your health and quality of life, six hours or less per week should suffice while you pursue a well-balanced life. An outline of the proposed exercise program follows the suggested weight-training guidelines. Foremost is the Principle of Moderation.

Lifting Technique

Your workout objectives dictate the lifting technique you should use. For example, strength and power are of paramount importance to *competitive weight lifters* in preparing the muscles they use in their competitive lifts. This means they might favor slow, deliberate movements for short sets and heavy weights causing them to bulk up significantly. They will work on their explosive forces by practicing the actual lifts they use in competition.

Bodybuilders, interested in muscle size with symmetry and definition, will target specific muscles with steady, uniform movements that stress them in very precise directions. Using momentum by pulling hard on a weight would be considered "cheating," because it engages other muscles to assist the one being isolated (generally speaking, bodybuilders avoid multimuscle techniques).

Since my program aims to stress and vascularize as much muscle mass as possible to reduce blood pressure effectively, I recommend using enough *controlled momentum* to engage other muscles in addition to the targeted muscle. The exercise then becomes a multimuscle effort. Do this for every set *not* marked **S**. Do not lift the weights explosively! Because you are bringing more muscles into play when you lift with momentum, you can use a heavier weight for these exercises, but you must avoid twisting the lower back during any lift! Do wait until the end of the *initial six weeks* before using controlled momentum.

Initial Six Weeks

And what weight should you start with? Lighter or heavier? Be safe—and patient. Start with the lighter weight (say, one that you can easily do twenty repetitions with). For the first six weeks or so of the program outlined below, do three ten-rep sets for all of the exercises listed. Apply the Progressive Overload Principle for these weeks, increasing the weight slightly every two weeks or so—*but without going to failure yet*. After six weeks or so, switch to the Principle of Moderation by following the guidelines provided below.

Principle of Moderation (M)

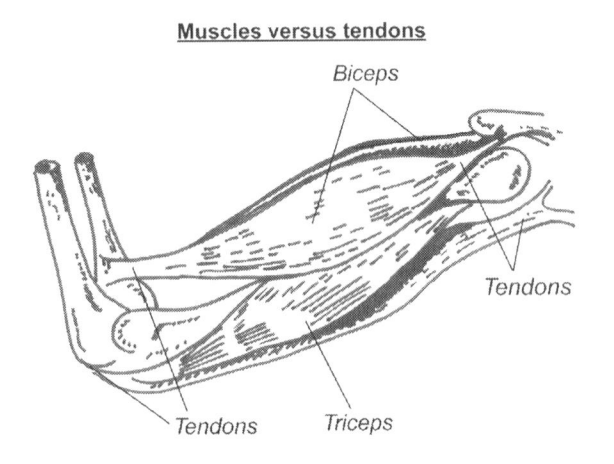

Muscles, due to their superior blood supply, strengthen much faster than their tendons in response to weight-training intensity. Hence, a sudden, strong contraction by a strengthened muscle might strain and injure its weaker, unprepared tendon and cause a long-term injury. Tendons and ligaments, due to their meager blood supply, heal very slowly. This could interfere with your goal of long-term participation and thus with achieving your fitness objectives. The *Principle of Moderation* (see Heart of the Program below for its application) is designed to counter this danger by making the lifter use the same weight for a longer period after the muscle has reached its peak strength for that resistance. Using the same resistance for a few extra weeks means the muscle's increased strength *stays the same* as it "waits" for the strength of its tendons and ligaments to catch up (adapt). This diminishes the risk of injury.

The Heart of the Program—Exercises Marked M for Moderation

For all exercises marked **M**, start with the weight you've attained at the end of your initial six-week period. Do ten reps *for the first and second sets only*, but start trying to reach fifteen reps for the *third set*. This will probably require two or more weeks. Once you can do fifteen reps for the third set consistently (say, for two or three more sessions), increase the weight for the *first set of ten reps* by five pounds (or less) for the ensuing sessions.

For the next sessions continue with the original weight for the second and third sets, again trying for fifteen reps in the third. The fact that you have increased the first set weight will tire you enough to prevent you from again doing fifteen reps during your third set. You may require a few weeks of going to failure before you can get back to doing fifteen reps for the third set. Once you can do fifteen consistently, augment the *second set's* weight by five pounds (or less) for ensuing sessions. Do not change the third-set weight yet! Again try to reach fifteen reps for the third set (this may take you a while, as before).

Once you can do fifteen reps consistently with the original third-set weight, raise the *third-set weight* by five pounds (or less) for the following sessions. Again, using the new weight, try to get to fifteen reps for the third set. When you can do this, raise the first-set weight by another five pounds (or less), and so on.

Keep repeating the pattern. This way, your strength improves gradually over the months at a rate more amenable to the development of your tendons and ligaments. Meanwhile, you are always *lifting to failure* for the third set, which is important for vascularization!

Remember that returning the weight slowly to its starting position at the end of a rep (the negative rep) is also a very effective way to strengthen tendons and ligaments.

Different Angles

Exercises marked **M** are followed by a variety of other exercises, all aimed at working the same muscle but at somewhat different angles. Stressing different parts of the same muscle vascularizes and develops it more effectively (Chapter 13). You should also try to increase the weight for these exercises according to the Progressive Overload Principle. For all of these exercises not marked **M**, change to a weight that lets you reach failure at ten reps or so at the end of the *initial six weeks*. For the sake of strengthening tendons and ligaments, continue with that weight for a few more sessions before you increase to a weight that now gives you failure at seven or eight reps. Carry on with that new weight until you again get to ten reps or so three or four weeks later. Use this weight for a few more sessions (again for the tendons and ligaments), then progressively increase the weight again. Keep repeating this pattern.

Strict Repetitions—Exercises Marked S

A *strict* repetition is one where the weight is raised slowly during the concentric part of the lift and returned slowly to its original position during its eccentric part. In the program outlined below, sets of strict reps marked **S** usually come after the muscle has been prefatigued by prior controlled-momentum exercises. You might need to reduce the weight used for the strict sets. This technique not only exhausts the muscles further for more effective vascularization; it also strengthens the tendons and ligaments during the negative rep part of the lift.

Rest Periods

During the initial six weeks of your weight-training program, rest three minutes between sets, and six minutes between each muscle worked. Shorten these rest periods gradually to two and five minutes as your fitness level improves (say, after ten weeks or so). The longer rest periods are included in the following outline.

The Program

SESSION 1 – Monday

Warm-up

No rest

Biceps

a) Biceps Curls (cable machine)—**M** for 3 sets. Stand up, facing the cable machine.

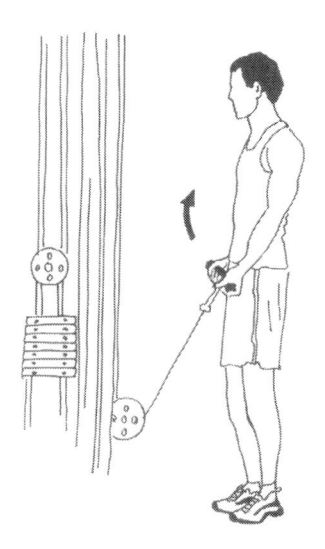

Starting position 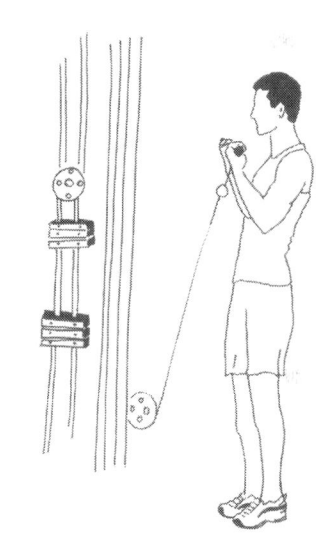 **Direction and range of lift**

b) Preacher Curls (with EZ bar)—2 sets of 10. Using an undergrip on an EZ bar, sit with arms on the preacher bench.

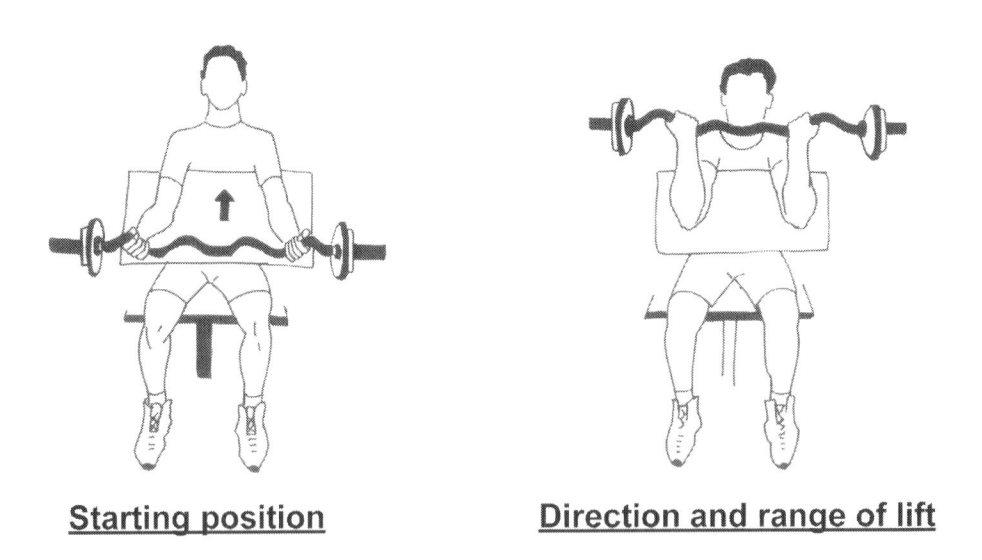

Starting position   **Direction and range of lift**

c) Sitting Dumbbell Biceps Curls—1 set of 20. Alternate arms.

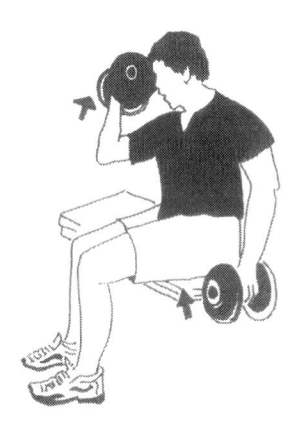

Alternate arms

d) Pull-ups—With hands facing in**,** go to failure each time.

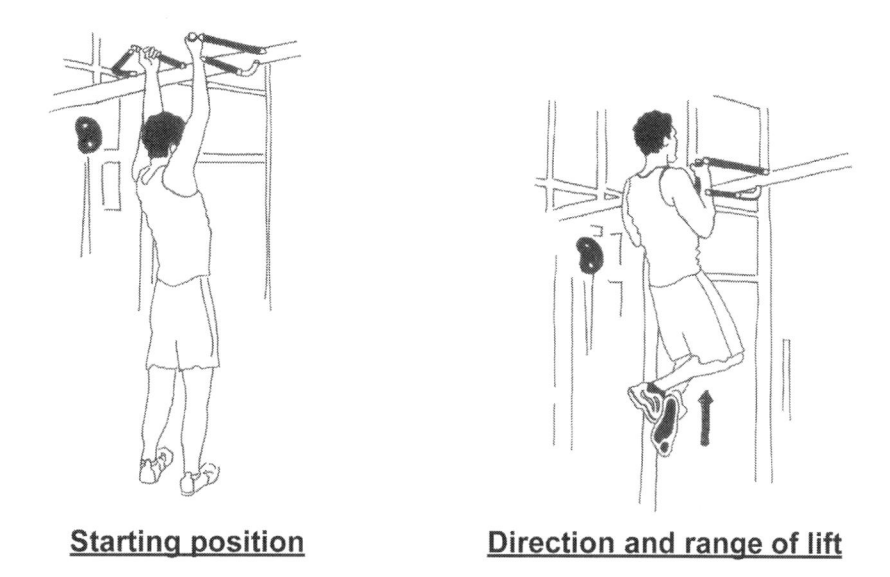

Starting position   **Direction and range of lift**

e) Barbell Curls—2 **S** sets of 10 (pyramid down). Stand up and use a straight barbell.

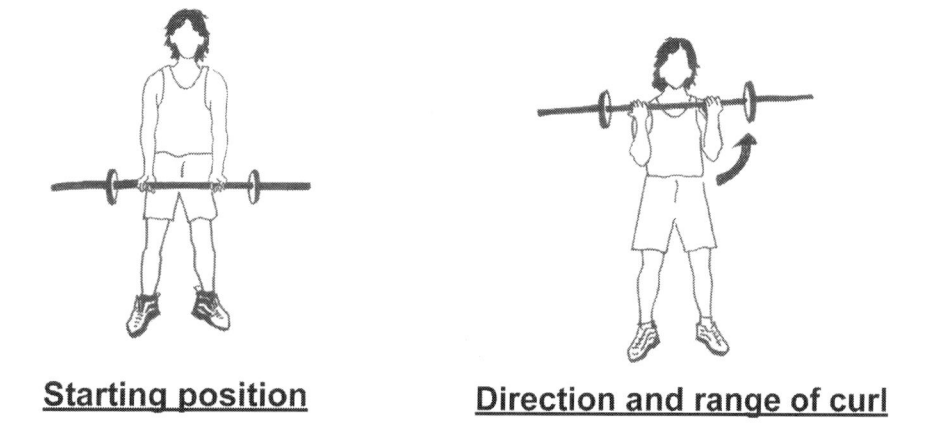

Starting position   **Direction and range of curl**

f) Rest 5 minutes.

Quadriceps

a) Leg Press Machine—4 sets: 3 sets of 10 leg presses (pyramid down). **S** for the 4th set.

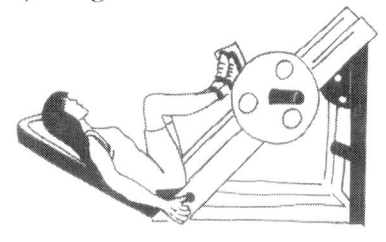

Starting position 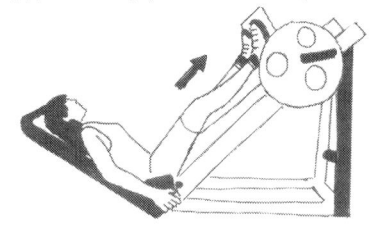   **Direction and range of push**

b) Leg Extension Machine—**S** for 2 sets of 10.

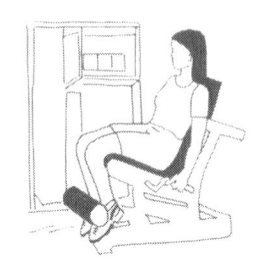

Starting position 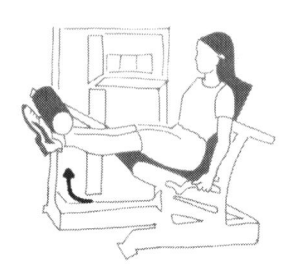   **Direction and range of lift**

Hamstrings

Hamstring Machine—3 sets of 10 leg flexions (pyramid down).

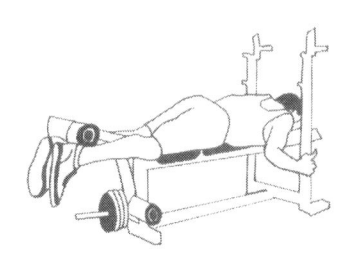

Starting position 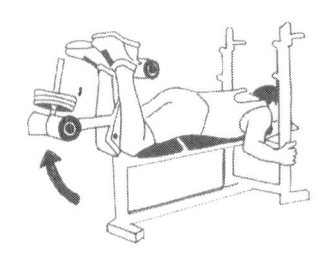   **Direction and range of the flexion**

Cardiovascular

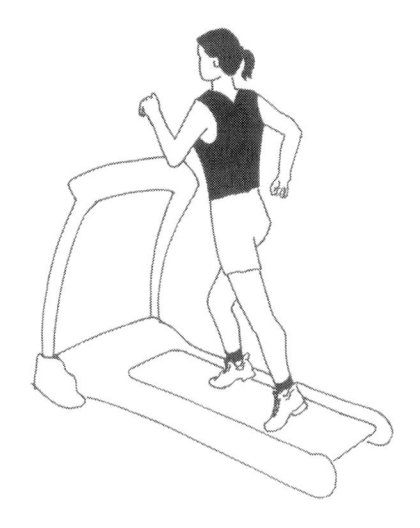

a) 15 to 25 minutes on the treadmill.

b) No rest.

Concentration and Hand-Eye Coordination

a) Use the speed bag (or any other such exercise, such as a skipping rope) for 7 or 8 minutes.

b) Rest a few minutes.

Mobility and Cool-Down

10 minutes of simple gymnastics, martial arts, or other movement, if you have the time.

SESSION 2 – Wednesday

Warm-up

No rest

Triceps

a) Pushdowns (cable machine)—**M** for 3 sets.

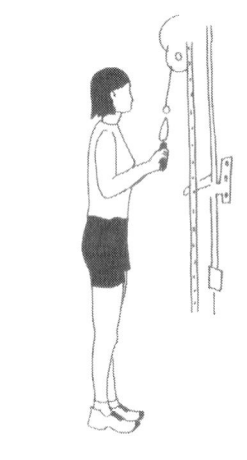

Starting position 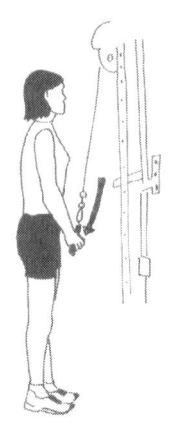   **Direction and range of push**

b) Dips—2 sets. Face the opposite direction for the second set if the bars angle out. Build up to 15 reps, then increase the resistance by hanging weights from a waist belt.

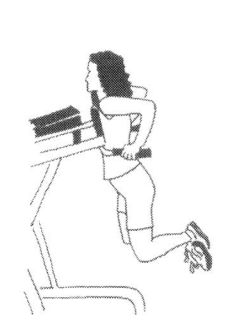

Starting position 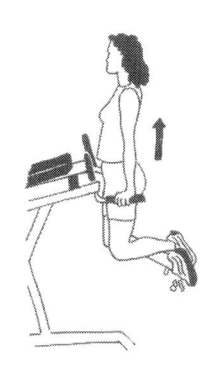   **Direction and range of push**

c) Kickbacks—2 sets of 10 with each arm (pyramid down). One-knee kneel on a bench with back horizontal.

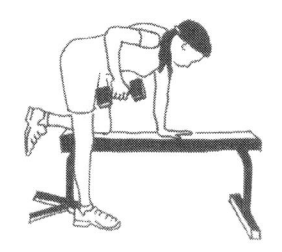

Starting position 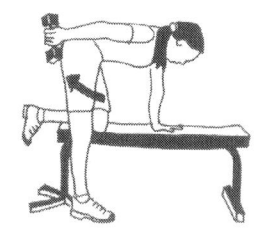   **Direction and range of lift**

d) Arm Extension on Preacher's Bench—2 sets of 10. Use an overgrip with hands angled.

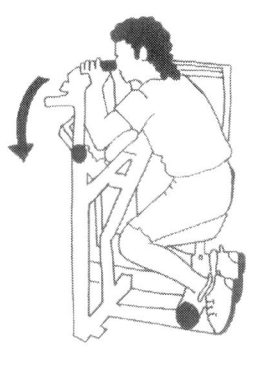

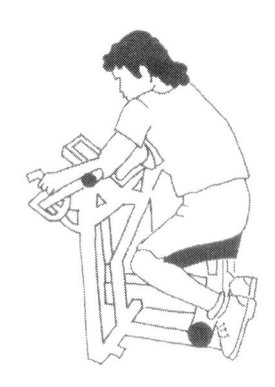

Starting position **Range of push down**

e) Rest 5 minutes.

You may already know that the bench press and the overhead press also work the triceps directly along with the targeted muscles (respectively pectorals and deltoids). Hence, the triceps are worked out often and quite intensively. Consider this when, for example, your commitments prevent you from doing your complete workout during a certain week. Simply leave out this triceps part of your regimen.

Back

a) Rowing Machine—4 sets: **M** for 3 sets + **S** for 1 set. For back safety, chest on the support pad is mandatory!

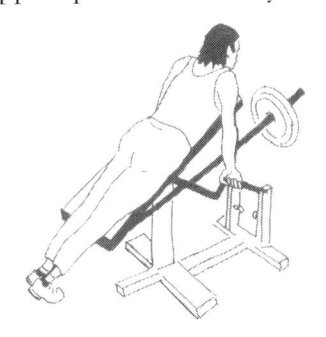

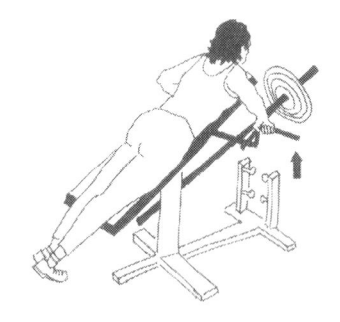

Starting position **Direction and range of lift**

b) Reverse Pull-Ups—1 set. Always go to failure. Start with 1 or 2 reps per session. Build up to 10 or more over the months.

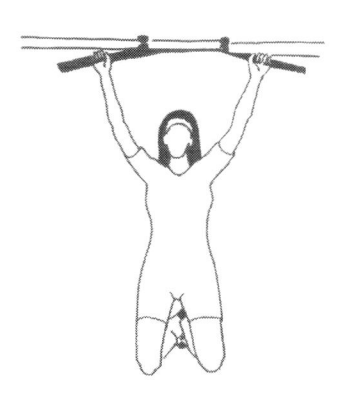

Starting position 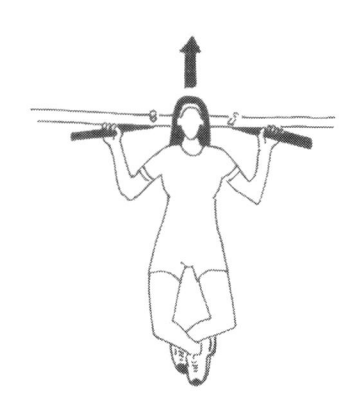   **Direction and range of lift**

c) Pull-Down Machine—2 sets of 20 reps each. For each set, alternate pulling the bar down to the chest while leaning back and then to just behind the top of the head with the upper body held vertically. *Pyramid* down for the second set.

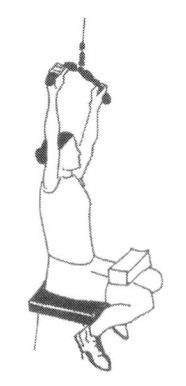

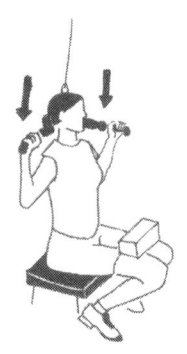

Starting position   **Direction and range of pull-down**

d) Reverse Flies on the Pec Dec Machine—1 set of 15. Sit down facing the machine and pull grips backward. Start with a heavier weight and pause to drop the weight down during the set if you wish.

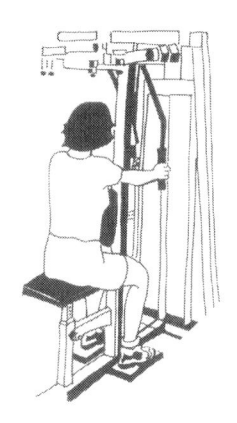

Starting position 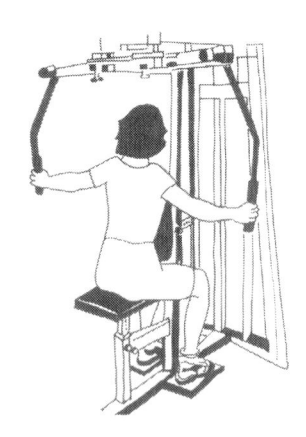   **Direction and range of pull**

e) Reverse Dumbbell Flies at 45 degrees—2 sets of 10 for the middle traps. *Pyramid* down for the second set.

Lie face down on the long bench, inclined at 45 degrees, and let the dumbbells hang straight down. Do each rep by raising the weights up vertically as high as you can with straight arms and hold momentarily. Contract the middle trapezius in the process. Stronger and hence *shorter* traps pull the scapulae back to the midline of the upper back chronically to help avoid shoulder impingement problems.

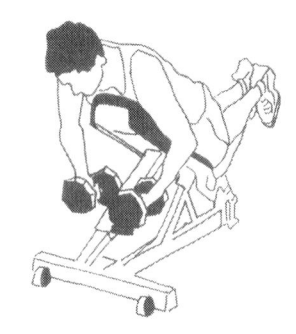

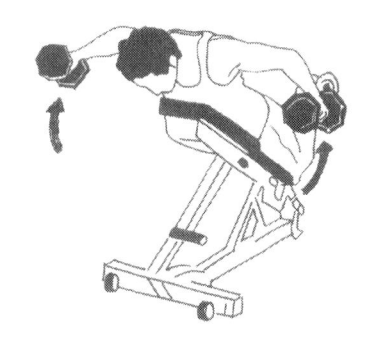

Starting position   **Direction and range of the side lifts**

Rest 5 minutes.

Cardiovascular

a) 15 to 25 minutes on the treadmill.

b) No rest.

Concentration and Hand-Eye Coordination

c) Use the speed bag (or any other such exercise, such as a skipping rope) for 7 or 8 minutes.

d) Rest a few minutes.

Mobility and Cool-Down

10 minutes of simple gymnastics, martial arts, or other movement, if you have the time.

SESSION 3 – Friday

Warm-up

No rest

Shoulders

a) Overhead Press Machine—4 sets: **M** for 3 sets + **S** for 1 set.

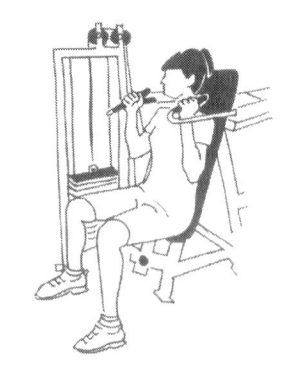

Starting position 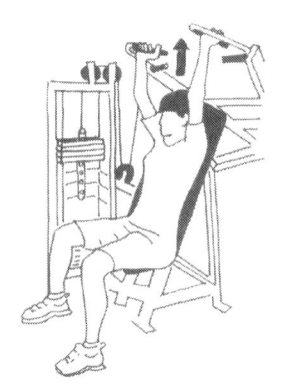 **Direction and range of press**

b) Upright Rowing with barbell—2 sets of 12 (pyramid down). Bar starts at waist with hands less than shoulder width apart; lift the bar up to the chin.

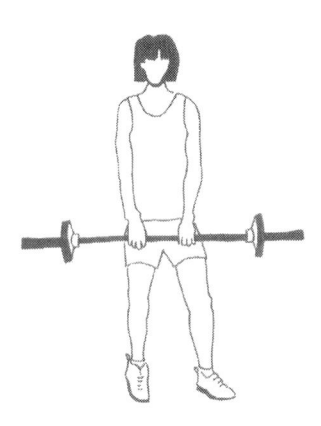

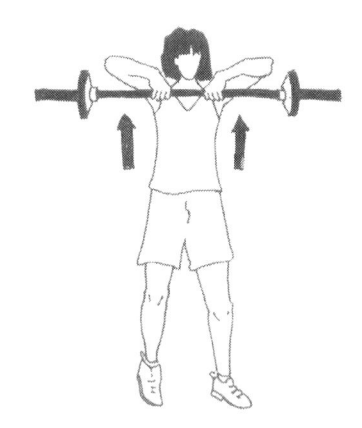

Starting position **Direction and range of lift**

c) Side Laterals with dumbbells (standing)—2 sets of 12 (pyramid down).

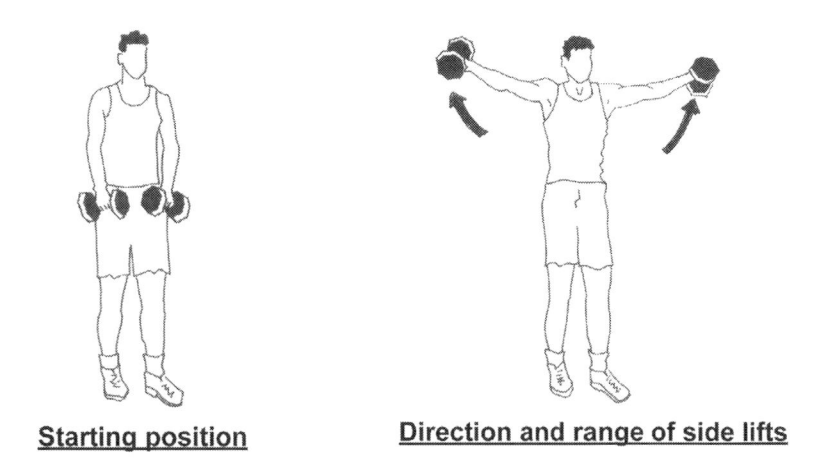

Starting position   **Direction and range of side lifts**

d) Overhead Press with barbell—1 set. Using a wider-than-shoulder-width grip, alternate down to the front of the head and to the top of the back of the head. (This gives the medial deltoids a more balanced workout.). Progressively overload.

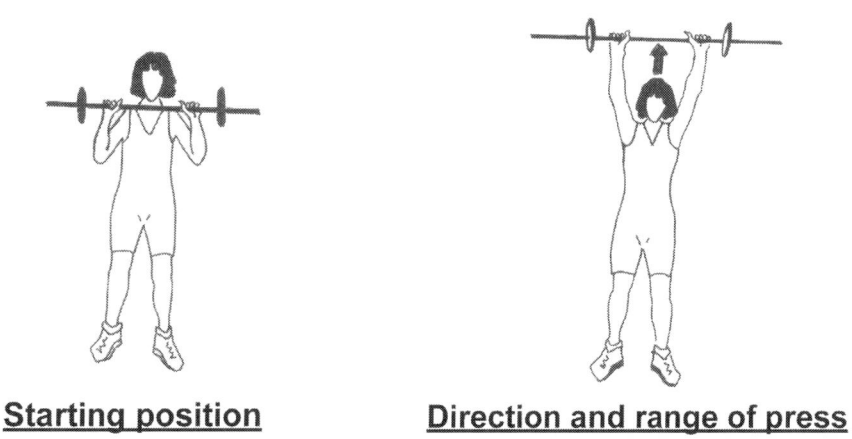

Starting position   **Direction and range of press**

e) Rest 5 minutes.

Chest

a) Bench Press—4 sets: **M** for 3 sets + **S** for 1 set.

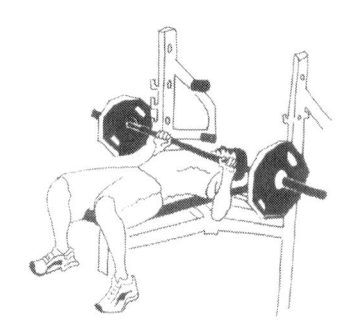

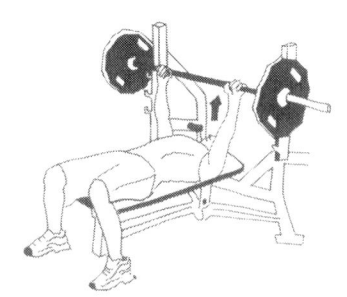

Starting position   **Direction and range of press**

b) Flies—1 set of 20 reps on the Pec Dec machine: alternate arms. Use full range of movement for each arm by rotating the gripping hand to the *opposite* shoulder.

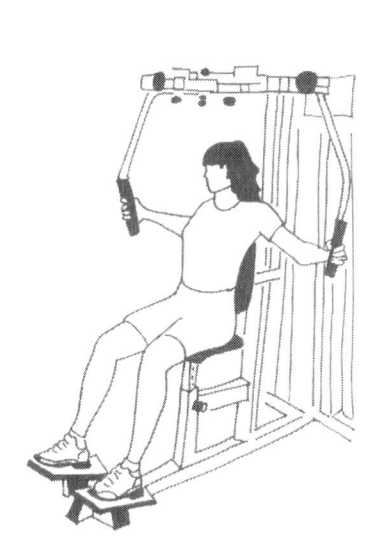

Starting position

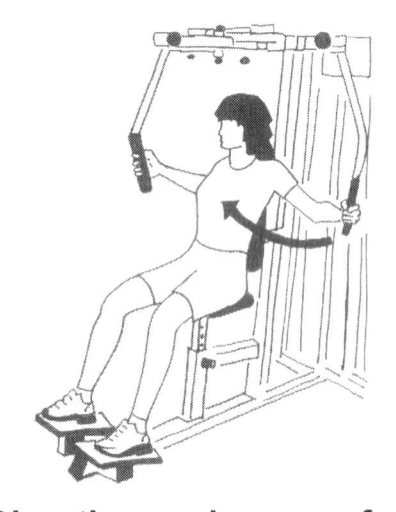

Direction and range of pull
Left hand to right shoulder
Right hand to left shoulder

c) Dumbbell Incline Press (head higher than knees)—2 sets of 10 (*pyramid* down for the second set).

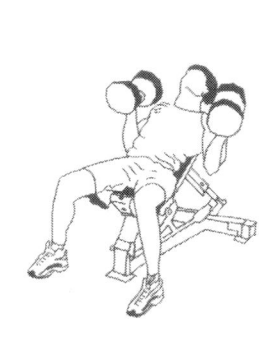

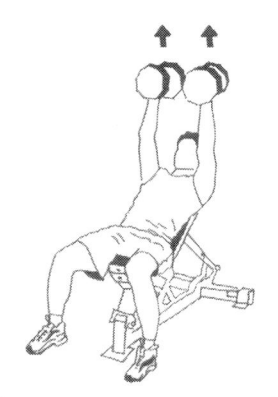

Starting position   **Direction and range of press**

d) Barbell Decline Press (head lower than knees)—3 sets of 10 (*pyramid* down for the second and third sets).

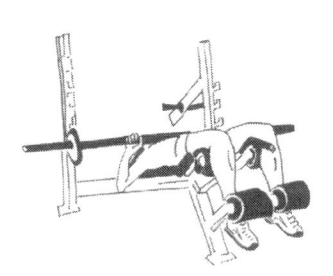

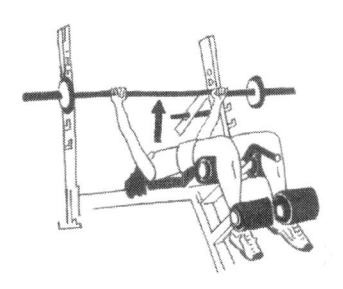

Starting position   **Direction and range of press**

e) Rest 5 minutes.

Cardiovascular

a) 15 to 25 minutes on the treadmill.

b) No rest.

Concentration and Hand-Eye Coordination

a. Use the speed bag (or any other such exercise, such as a skipping rope) for 7 or 8 minutes.

b. Rest a few minutes.

Mobility and Cool-Down

10 minutes of simple gymnastics, martial arts, or other movement, if you have the time.

I use this program with the equipment available at my gym, and it gives me the desired results. The longer you follow this program, the more you will understand your body and its capabilities. You are certainly free to alter the program according to your available equipment and time, your capabilities, and your preferences, as long as you adhere to the basic principles explained throughout *Reduce Blood Pressure through Weight Training*.

CHAPTER 18

IS YOUR PROGRAM WORKING? AND AFTERTHOUGHTS

It is not difficult to tell if your fitness program is improving your strength and flexibility: you can lift more weight and stretch farther as you proceed from one month to the next. But please do not forget to apply the five practical and reliable tests listed below to determine if you are working hard enough to achieve the important health benefits you want; they will also tell you if you are spending more time in the gym than needed. Vague tests with *vague results* might cause you to spend more time than necessary working out in the gym, thereby preventing you from pursuing other interests that enrich your life. As a result, sadly, because the real key to success is *consistent long-term participation*, you might quit your program prematurely.

Give yourself the chance to experience the changes in strength and endurance I know you can achieve. Follow your program with adequate intensity for an adequate time (at least eight months). Once you see the results, I'm sure you'll keep going.

Run my five tests regularly:

1. Take your resting pulse rate (see Chapter 1 for details)
2. Take your resting blood pressure (see Chapter 6 for details).
3. Measure your waist (see Chapter 10 for details).
4. Weigh yourself (see Chapter 10 for details).
5. Calculate your waist-hip ratio (see Chapter 10 for details).

Consider the following factors as you are interpreting the results:

Athletic Ability

Some people who consider themselves nonathletic think only a "real" athlete can lower resting pulse rate or achieve any of the other objectives I list. Nothing could be further from the truth. The deciding factors for success are the intensity of a workout and adherence to it. Anybody, athletically inclined or not, *can train with the proper intensity*.

While at Work

Many fitness books provide guidelines for fitness activities at work. This is commendable, but I don't think you get a proper workout that way. Set time aside to use suitable resistance in a gym where the environment is more conducive to demanding effort. If you train with focus and intensity, you'll reach your objectives.

Older Individuals

Individuals over fifty are quite capable of intensity in their workouts. Just like anyone, they can gradually adapt to sensible physical discomfort. Of course, they have to check with their health-care provider prior to starting a program. The simple tests I propose can motivate anyone to build up to the intensity that produces rewarding results.

You can improve your strength at any age

APPENDIX A

MY PERSONAL RESEARCH RECORD: INTERPRETATION AND ASSESSMENT

The monthly averages of my readings taken since February 2008 are below, with (at times) relevant notes about my physical condition and/or location. I took seventy to ninety readings per sitting for about twenty sittings per month.

- Feb. 2008—160/81
- Mar. 2008—151/68
- April 2008—150/76
- May 2008—148/74
- June 2008—136/70
- July 2008—130/70
- Aug. 2008—127/68 (moderately heavy weight lifting)
- Sept. 2008—other commitments
- Oct. 2008—127/65 (moderately heavy weight lifting)

- Nov. 2008—115/61 (heavy weight lifting)
- Dec. 2008—119/60 (started lifting to failure)
- Jan. 2009—117/59 (lifting to failure with heavier weights)
- Feb. 2009—first 2 weeks—117/60 (lifting to failure with heavy weights)
- Feb. 2009—last 2 weeks—bad cold
- Mar. 2009—1st week—cold ending
- Mar. 2009—2nd week—128/63
- Mar. 2009—3rd week—114/58
- April 2009—first 3 weeks—bronchitis
- April 2009—last week—115/61 (back to heavy weight lifting)
- May 2009—115/58 (experimenting with heavier weight training)
- June 2009—1st week—115/59 (experimenting with heavier weights)
- June 2009—2nd and 3rd week—vacationing in the Adirondacks
- June 2009—4th week—114/59 (experimenting with heavier weights)
- August 2009—1st week 115/59
- August 2009—2nd and 3rd week—Nova Scotia vacation
- September 2009—116/62
- October 2009—1st and 2nd weeks—118/59
- October 2009—3rd week—respite
- October 2009—4th week—120/59 (heavier weights)
- November 2009—119/59—extrahard workouts; vaccinated on Nov. 27
- December 2009—124/62—3 sessions per week (with a 2nd week respite)
- January 2010—120/60—3 tough sessions per week
- February 2010—1st week—119/59
- February 2010—2nd week—ill with flu
- February 2010—3rd and 4th week—118/57
- March 2010—118/58—strenuous workouts
- April 2010—121/55—strenuous workouts
- May 2010—120/55—very strenuous workouts
- June 2010—116/55—very strenuous workouts
- July 2010—113/52—very strenuous workouts
- September 2010—118/58—medium-intensity workouts
- October 2010—116/55—medium-intensity workouts

- November 2010—111/51—regular workouts
- December 2010—113/53—regular workouts first 3 weeks
- January 2011—115/53—regular workouts
- February 2011—no readings, irregular workouts
- March 2011—116/53—regular workouts
- April 2011—117/54—very strenuous workouts
- May 2011—114/53—very strenuous workouts
- June 2011—113/52—very strenuous workouts
- July 2011—no readings; no workouts
- August 2011—no readings; light to heavy workouts
- September 2011—114/52—regular workouts
- October 2011—114/53—regular workouts

My workouts during these months were moderately intensive to very strenuous. By about November 2011, I noticed that my readings were quite low, but my health was fine; *I was never dizzy, and definitely not weak.* I had had a November 2010 reading of *67/42* and one in December 2010 of *63/44*. Many systolic readings were in the 80s and 90s, and some in the 70s. Curious, I tried a second, identical monitor, but it gave readings in the same low range. Meanwhile, I had sent the first monitor back to the company that manufactured it for verification; they said its calibration was 100 percent accurate.

My monitor gives *error* readings EE when the diastolic result is below *40*; I obtained hundreds of such readings that could therefore not be recorded along with their corresponding systolic figures. It seemed as though the harder I worked, the more my systolic and diastolic results dropped. To achieve normotensive (115/75) results, much less effort is required.

Such low blood pressure values, resulting from perfectly acceptable anatomical changes to the circulatory system in response to the unique training principles I outline, are certainly desirable.

I obtained these results with workouts three times per week: weight training for an hour and a half and brisk walking on a treadmill for twenty-five minutes. **The walking component alone would not have given me these superb results.**

Although these are not the results of a *properly designed* cross-sectional experiment, because I was the only test subject, it is difficult to refute what so many readings over a three-year period imply. I certainly welcome—and look forward to—the results of more rigorous, peer-reviewed scientific scrutiny. I am sure that research will support my contention that weight training can very effectively reduce blood pressure.

APPENDIX B

ONE-SITTING READINGS FROM NOVEMBER 26TH, 2010

Please take special note of highs and lows of the systolic and diastolic ranges for each set.

	SYS	DIA	
Average of all data	102	53	
Time	SYS	DIA	Special event
15:38	118	57	Started half hour after
15:38	116	58	very strenuous workout
15:37	120	63	
15:36	109	49	
15:35	99	44	
15:34	108	45	
15:33	102	48	
15:33	90	56	
15:32	106	47	

Time	SYS	DIA
15:32	113	42
15:31	104	40
15:30	87	52
15:30	119	60
15:29	110	45
15:27	89	56
Time	SYS	DIA
15:27	106	41
15:26	87	49
15:25	85	51
15:25	67	42
15:24	93	45
15:23	119	58
15:23	82	59
15:22	108	49
15:21	112	47
15:20	117	48
15:20	92	52
15:19	93	51
15:18	100	47
15:18	96	49
15:17	110	48
15:17	109	51
15:16	113	73
15:15	105	46
15:14	102	48
15:13	91	59
15:13	107	68
15:12	101	54
15:11	100	54
15:11	106	48
15:10	110	45
15:09	93	56

Time	SYS	DIA
15:08	120	47
15:08	107	55
15:07	122	50
15:06	105	54
15:06	95	49
15:05	116	52
Time	SYS	DIA
15:04	87	41
15:04	120	50
15:03	98	49
15:02	119	49
15:02	98	61
15:01	104	57
15:00	77	58
15:00	100	56
14:59	105	76
14:58	99	64
14:57	96	71
14:57	99	79
14:56	88	51
14:55	118	42
14:54	88	68
14:53	113	56
14:52	121	56
14:51	85	56
14:50	103	67

References

Each of the references shown below provides an expanded source of information for some detail or details given in the related section (preface, chapter, etc.). These sources can be accessed by using the web address given or, if that is not available or does not function, by Googling the title and associated information such as authors' names and date published.

Every effort has been made to trace the copyright holders, but any who have been overlooked are invited to get in touch with the publishers (or the author)

Preface

American Heart Association. "Preventive Health Care - Why is preventive health care so important?" Sept. 7, 2009.

Harvard Medical School. "Ten ways to lower blood pressure." Sept. 2006. http://www.health.harvard.edu/press_releases/lower-blood-pressure.

Heart and Stroke Foundation of Canada. "High blood pressure: Canada's crisis in the making." Feb 18, 2010. http://www.cbc.ca/technology/high-blood-pressure-canada-8-crisis-in-the-making-1.871223

Tanner, Lindsay. "Blood pressure goal met: Half of afflicted Americans control it with medication." May 25, 2010. Sympatico.ca http://www.nhlbi.nih.gov/health/dci/Diseases/Hbp/HBP_Whatis.html.

Introduction

Pavey, T., N. Anokye, A. Taylor, P. Trueman, T. Moxham, et al. "'Weak evidence' to support exercise referrals." NIHR Health Technology Assessment 2011; 15(44). http://www.journalslibrary.nihr.ac.uk/hta/volume- 15/issue-44.

Tobin, Anne-Marie. "The ups and downs of weight loss: Success not always measured on the scale." Mar. 3, 2010. Sympatico. ca.

Chapter 1

Editors of Men's Health. "Lower your heart rate to prevent a heart attack." Feb. 5, 2010. http://www.nbc.news.com/id/33451255/ns/health-heart_health/t/lower-your...

World Health Organization. "Mean Systolic Blood Pressure." http://www.who.int/gho/ncd/risk_factors/blood_pressure_mean_text/en/.

Chapter 2

Meier, P., H. Hemingway, A. J. Lansky, G. Knapp, B. Pitt, C. Seiler. "The impact of the coronary collateral circulation on mortality: a meta-analysis." European Heart Journal, 2011. DOI: 10.1093/eurheartj/ehr308.

Miller, Joe. "Does exercise increase red blood cells?" Sept. 3, 2011. http://www.livestrong.com/article/534560-does-exercise-increase-red-blood-cells.

Kathiresan, Sekar. "Plasma HDL cholesterol and risk of myocardial infarction: A mendelian randomisation study." Lancet, Aug. 11, 2012. http://www.thelancet.com/journals/lancet/article/PIISO140-6736%2812%.

Chapter 3

Krustrup, Peter, Ylva Hellsten, and Jens Bangsbo. "Intense interval training enhances human skeletal muscle uptake in the initial phase of dynamic exercise at high but not at low intensities." http://www.ncbi.nlm.nih.gov/pmc/articles/PMC1665058/.

Chapter 5

Harvard Medical School. "Ten ways to lower blood pressure." Sept. 2006. http://www.health.harvard.edu/press_releases/lower-blood-pressure.

Srikanthan, Preethi and Arun Karlamangla. "Increased muscle mass may lower risk of diabetes." Journal of Clinical Endocrinology & Metabolism, July 28, 2011.

Chapter 7

Branswell, Helen. "Expect the unexpected: Cdn kids' blood pressure not up, despite obesity rates." Sympatico.ca. May 19, 2010.

Carlson, Dusten. "Massachusetts sends parents 'Hey, your kids are fat' letters." Feb. 26, 2013. http://www.inquisitr.com/545337/massachusetts-sends-parents-hey-your-kids-are-fat-letters

"Waist-hip ratio best predictor of heart attack risk." Nov. 4th, 2004. Based on an Interheart study by Dr. Salim Yusuf and Dr. Arya Sharmaa of McMaster University and published in The Lancet.

Chapter 11

Tanner, Lindsey. "No wonder you've got middle-aged spread: Women need hour of exercise a day to keep it off." Sympatico.ca. Mar. 23, 2010.

Yang, K., H. Guan, E. Arany, D. J. Hill, X. Cao. "Neuropeptide Y is produced in visceral adipose tissue and promotes proliferation of adipocyte precursor cells via the Y1 receptor." The FASEB Journal 22, (2008): 2452-2464.

Chapter 16

American Heart Association. "Regular physical activity reduces risk of dementia in older people." Nov. 1, 2012. http://newsroom.heart.org/pr/aha/_prv-regular-physical-activity-reduces-240181.aspx

Neergaard, Lauran. "Study will put to test growing evidence linking high blood pressure to dementia." Sympatico.ca. Jan. 25, 2010.

Srikanthan, Preethi and Arun Karlamangla. "Increased muscle mass may lower risk of diabetes." Journal of Clinical Endocrinology & Metabolism, July 28, 2011.

Ubelacker, Sheryl. "Weight training improves seniors' cognitive abilities: Research." Sympatico.ca. Jan. 25, 2010.

Chapter 18

Marshall, P.W. and I. Desai. "Electromyographic analysis of upper body, lower body, and abdominal muscles during advanced Swiss ball exercises." http://www.ncbi.nlm.nih.gov/pubmed/20508456.

Suggested Readings

Many thanks to the authors for their enlightening information.

Anderson, Bob, Bill Pearl, Ed Burke, and Jeff Galloway. *Getting Back in Shape: 32 Workout Programs for Lifelong Fitness.* 3rd ed. Bolinas, CA: Shelter Publications, 2007.

Cannon, Christopher P., MD, and Elizabeth Vierck. 2009. *The New Heart Disease Handbook: Everything You Need to Know to Effectively Reverse and Manage Heart Disease.* Beverly, MA: Fair Winds Press, 2009.

Mohrman, David E. and Lois Jane Heller. *Cardiovascular Physiology.* 7th ed. New York: McGraw-Hill Medical, 2010.

Smith, Denise L. and Bo Fernhall. *Advanced Cardiovascular Exercise Physiology.* Champaign, IL: Human Kinetics, 2011.

Delavier, Frédéric. *Strength Training Anatomy.* 3rd ed. Champaign, IL: Human Kinetics, 2010.

Kilavora, Peter. *Foundations of Exercise Science: Studying Human Movement and Health.* 2nd ed. Toronto: Sport Books Publisher, 2007.

Plowman, Sharon and Denise L. Smith. *Exercise Physiology for Health, Fitness and Performance.* 3rd ed. Philadelphia: Wolters Kluwer Health/Lippincott Williams & Wilkins, 2011. **PG**

Temertzoglou, Ted and Paul Challen. *Exercise Science: An Introduction to Health and Physical Education.* Toronto: Thompson Educational Publishing Inc., 2003.

Moore, Thomas MD, et al. *The DASH Diet for Hypertension: Lower Your Blood Pressure in 14 Days—Without Drugs.* New York: Pocket Books, 2001.

Index

Cross-referencing integrated throughout the index should facilitate the search for information.

Adequate intensity,
    why necessary, xiv, 14, 23, 73,

Adherence,
    and athletic ability, 128,
    definition, xiv,
    for discipline, perseverance, and tenacity, 103,
    for success, xiv,
    info encouraging adherence, chapter 7,
    see also diminishing returns,

Adhesions,
    definition, 76,
    post-exercise soreness, 76,

Aerobic energy,
    and dynamic resistance activity, 19,
    definition, 19,

Aerobics (cardiovascular),
    exercises for, 48,
    loss of muscle mass, 62,

Age and,
    functionality, 101,
    hardening of the arteries (arteriosclerosis), 9,
    sarcopenia, 101,

Agonist muscle,
    muscle tone and postural considerations, 88,
    opposing muscles, 88,
    role in movement, 88,
    role reversal, 88,

Agility,
    enhancement, 103,

Anaerobic energy,
    and dynamic resistance activity, 19,
    definition, 19,

Anatomical changes,
    acquired at what pace, xv
    desired changes, xv,

Angiogenesis,
    and blood pressure, 31,
    and hypertrophied muscle, 31,
    definition, 31,

Antagonist muscle,
    muscle tone and postural considerations, 88,
    opposing muscles, 88,
    role in movement, 88,
    role reversal, 88,

Antiarrythmic drugs,
    palliative therapeutic technique, xiii,

Aorta,
    and cardiovascular health, 24, 26,
    and diastolic pressure, 8
    atrophy, possibility of, 44
    definition, 8,
    force of contraction, 14, 23,
    see also windkessel effect,

Appetite and,
    hunger, 66
    NPY, 66,

Arteries,
    description and function, 3, 5, 13,
    increasing lumen diameter, 15,
    see also arteriosclerosis,
    see also atherosclerosis

Arterioles,
    and capillary density, 14,
    description and function, 5,
    see also vasoconstrict,
    see also vasodilate,

Arteriosclerosis,
    and blood pressure, 9-10,
    and cardiovascular exercises, 16,
    causes, 9,
    definition, 9,
    see also resistance,

Atherosclerosis,
    and blood pressure xiii, 9,
    and LDL cholesterol, 9, 15,
    and lumen size (illustrated), 9,
    and triglycerides, 9,
    and vascularisation, xiv,
    blockage, 10,
    cause, 8-9,
    clot formation, 10,
    definition, xiii, 9,
    see also arteries,
    see also endothelium,
    see also resistance,

Athletic ability,
    necessary?, 128,

Author,
    family and personal health history, xvii-xviii,
    formulating my rationale, xviii-xix, 39, 49,
    personal research record (monthly) 129-135,
    see also personal fitness program,

Back,
    anatomy of, 85,
    session 2 exercises, 118-120,
    multimuscle execises, 84-85,

Balloon angioplasty,
    palliative surgical technique, xiii,

Baseline reference value,
    resting blood pressure, 33-34,
    to monitor exercise program, 34,

Battery of tests,
    description, 45,
    limitations and valid alternative, 45-46,

Biceps,
    anatomy, 108,
    see also agonist,

Blood,
    its viscosity, 8
    oxygenated (red), 3,
    used (blue blood), 3,

Blood pressure,
    and increase in the lumen diameter of arteries, 15,
    and increased vascularisation of muscle mass, 30,
    and increasing capillary density, 14, 23,
    and milking action, 43
    and reducing the body's fat content, 15,
    dampening mechanisms during activity, 16, 43
    definition and purpose, 7-8,
    expressed in ratio form, 8,
    hypertensive (high), 8,
    measuring blood pressure, 10, 33-34,
    prehypertensive, 8, 10,
    risk of cardiovascular disease, 10,
    role of the heart and aorta, 8,
    see also diastolic blood pressure,
    see also resistance,
    see also systolic blood pressure,
    see also windkessel effect,
    when low values are acceptable, 131,
    when low values are not acceptable, 131,

Blood supply,
    greater volume of blood flow, 15,
    microcirculatory blood supply, 21,

Body mass index (BMI),
    calculation, 39,
    limitations, 39-40,
    validity versus waist-hip ratio, 40,
    versus waist-weight technique, 61-63,
    waist measurement adequate, 41,

Bodybuilding,
    health training regimen versus sport training regimen, 61,
    personal fitness program versus bodybuilding, 107,
    see also sports-oriented program,

Bones,
    and calcium, 102,
    see also osteoporosis,

Breathing while weight training,
    technique and purpose, 75,

Bulk up,
    large versus small muscles, 73,
    role of resistance, 14,
    see also hypertrophy,
    woman versus man xiv,

Calves,
    why not worked, 102,

Canadian Medical Association Journal,
    hypertension rates, xiii,

Capillaries,
    description and function, 5,
    resistance to blood flow, 23,
    rupture and its consequences, 10,

Capillary beds,
    description and function, 3, 5, 14,
    illustration, 4,

Capillary density,
    and flow rate, 14,
    and resistance to blood flow, 23
    and resting metabolic needs, 14,
    definition, 13-14,

how to increase capillary density, 13,
physiological benefits, 14-15,
see also vascularisation,

Cardiorespiratory endurance activities (or exercises),
and loss of muscle mass, 61, 62,
and muscle hypertrophy, 14,
effort required, 30,
limitations on blood pressure reduction, xiv, 29,
see also capillary density,
see also vascularization,
with weight training, 61,

Cardiovascular disease,
and average resting pulse, 44,
and increases in blood pressure, 10,
main risk factor xiii,
see also blood pressure – hypertensive and prehypertensive,
see also vascularisation,
shortcoming of palliative treatments xiii,

Cardiovascular health (or fitness),
advantages and limitations of cardiovascular training, 13, 29-30,
advantages of weight training, 29-30,
and brain development, 102,
high versus low intensity training, 102-103,
resting blood pressure, 102,
resting pulse rate, 102,
see also resistance to blood flow,

Cholesterol,
and atherosclerosis, 9, 15,
and damaged muscle cells, 67,
and hypertension, 15,
current research, 15,
HDL (happy) and LDL (lousy), 15,
impact of exercise on, 15,
see also resistance to blood flow,

Circulatory system,
arteries, 5,
arterioles, 5,
capillaries, 5,
capillary beds, 3,
general function, 5,
heart, 7,
milking action, 16,
response to activity, 3, 5, 6,
see also metabolite,
see also resistance to blood flow,
veins, 5,

Clot,
see also atherosclerosis,

Clot-busting drugs,
palliative therapy technique, xiii,

Concentric muscle contractions,
definition, 89,
and specificity, 89,

Contraction pattern of the heart,
and pulse rate, 24
description, 24,
see also heart,

Cool-down,
rationale, 104,
how, 104

Core circulation,
definition, 29,
see also peripheral circulation,

Crunches,
warm-up exercise, 101,
technique, 101,
abdominals and not iliopsoas (hip flexors), 101,
postural benefits to lower back, 101,

Detraining,
    definition, 77,
    consequences, 17, 77,

Diastolic blood pressure,
    and capillary density, 14, 30, 31, 33,
    and cardiovascular training, xiv, 29,
    and detraining, 77,
    and increased resistance to blood
        flow, 10,
    definition and ratio form expression, 8,
    neurogenic and biochemical controls, 26,
    pre-hypertensive and hypertensive
        levels, 10
    response to stress, 34,
    role of the aorta, 8, 23-26,
    see also windkessel effect,
    versus systolic pressure (MAP), 35

Diastole,
    calcium-releasing mechanism, 24,
    definition, 24,
    pressure gradient, 24,
    see also contraction pattern of the heart,
    zero ventricular pressure, 24,

Dieting,
    diet and behaviour guidelines, 57-59,
    dieting alone loses needed muscle mass,
        61,
    rule of thumb for daily calorie
        consumption, 58,

Different angles,
    rationale and procedure, 110,
    see also whole muscle training,
    training the whole muscle, 79-85,

Diminishing returns,
    advantage of understanding this concept,
        49,
    and competitive athletes, 49,

    definition, 49,
    deterrent to adherence, 49,
    see also adherence.

Doctors,
    exercises prescribed by, xix,

Eccentric muscle contraction,
    and specificity, 89,
    definition, 89,
    negative rep, 89,
    purpose (practicality), 89,

Endomorphic build,
    and BMI, 40,
    definition, 40,

Endothelial lesions,
    and atherosclerosis, 9,
    healing of lesions, 9,
    see also endothelium,
    see also atherosclerosis,
    causes, 8-9,
    definition, 8-9,
    and blood pressure, 9-16,

Endothelium,
    description, 8,
    see also endothelial lesions,

Extension,
    straightening a limb: ex. triceps extension,
        88,

Faddish fitness programs,
    limitations of Swiss exercise balls, 46,
    misleading expectations, 46,
    vascularisation? of skeletal muscle, 46,

Failure, muscular exhaustion,
    and maximum intensity, 74,
    and vasculartzation, 30,

cardiovascular benefits, xiv, 30, 43,
definition of failure, 30, 73, 74,
failure and individual strength, xiv, 102,
lactic acid as fatigue acid, 5, 6,
saturating the stressed muscle with lactic acid, 30,
see also fatigue acid,
see also lactic acid,
spotting, and lifting to failure, 74,
sprinting versus jogging, 30,
when to start going to failure, 73, 109, 110,

Fatigue acid,
see also lactic acid,

Fat content,
see also body mass index (BMI),
see also skinfold technique,
see also waist-weight procedure,
versus muscle content, 30, 61, 101,

Fitness programs,
see also health-oriented fitness program,
see also personal fitness program,
see also sports-oriented fitness program,

Flexion,
bending a limb: ex. biceps curl, 88,

Flow rate of blood,
and blood pressure, 8, 14,
and lumen size, 15,
and metabolic needs, 8, 14,
see also atherosclerosis,

Forearms,
why not worked, 102,

Functionality,
definition, 101,
see also health-oriented fitness program,

General objectives,
preface, xiii to xvi,
see also author,

Health-oriented fitness program,
components: warm-up and flexibility; strength and muscular endurance; cardiovascular fitness; concentration and hand-eye coordination; agility; discipline, perseverance, and tenacity, 100-104,
concentration and hand-eye coordination, 103,
discipline, perseverance, and tenacity, 103,
objectives, 99-100,
priorities, 11, 104,
see also agility,
see also cool-down,
see also functionality,
see also osteoporosis,

Heart attack,
cause, 10,
see also atherosclerosis,
see also cardiovascular disease,

Heart,
and hypertension, 42-44,
and its hypertrophy, 42-44,
atrophy, possibility of, 44,
contraction pattern, 24,
direction of blood flow, 7, 24,
force of contraction, 14, 23,
its parts (illustration), 7,
pulse rate, 24,
see also heart attack,
thickness of left ventricular wall, 7,
topping up the ventricles, 24,

Heart of the program,
lifting pattern after initial six weeks, 109,
lifting to failure, 110,

see also negative rep,

Heart rate,
    five monitoring tests, 44,
    heart rate reserve method, 44,
    resting pulse rate and resting blood pressure, 44,
    see also cardiovascular endurance activities,
    there is a better way, 44,
    to determine intensity levels, limitations, 44,

Homeostasis,
    cardiac pressure and aortic pressure in response to metabolic needs, 14, 23

Hypertension,
    and hypertrophy of the heart, 42-44,
    and vascularisation, xiv,
    body's response to hypertension, 10-11,
    definition, 8,
    imperceptible symptoms, the silent killer, 10,
    incidence and trends, xiii,
    need to take blood pressure, 10,
    pernicious, 42
    see also arteriosclerosis,
    see also atherosclerosis,
    see also resistance,
    weaknesses of the Public Health Agency of Canada's activity guidelines xiii,

Hypertensive blood pressure,
    definition, 8

Hypertrophy,
    definition, 42,
    see also bulk up,

Hypertrophy of skeletal muscle,
    and angiogenesis, 31,
    and blood pressure, 31,
    and capillary density, 31,
    and cardiovascular exercises, 14, 31,
    and resting metabolic needs, 31
    see also bulk up,
    see also hypertrophy,

Hypertrophy of the heart,
    a pathological condition, 42,
    and increased capillary density, 43-44,
    and isometric (static) weight training, 42-43,
    and isotonic weight training, 42-43,
    and marathon-like activities, 42,
    and pernicious hypertension, 42,
    atrophy, possibility of 44,
    dampening mechanisms, 43,
    exertion-induced increase in blood pressure, 43,
    heart and aorta contractions, 43-44,
    long-term overloading, 44,
    see also hypertrophy,

Initial six weeks,
    avoid excessive weight and going to failure, 108,
    see also personal fitness program,

Insertion of a muscle cell,
    definition, 81,
    role in movement, 81

Isometric contraction,
    advantage, 74,
    and hypertrophy of the heart, 42,
    definition, 74, 89,
    disadvantage: too much specificity, 74,

Isotonic contraction,
    and hypertrophy of the heart, 42-43,
    definition, 42, 74,
    see also muscle tone,

Insulin,
    insulin resistance and total muscle mass, 101

Intensity,
    enough to reduce resting pulse rate and blood pressure, 102,
    Rocky Balboa approach, xiv,
    stay with it for motivation, 127,

Journal of the American Medical Association,
    consequence of increases (and decreases) in blood pressure, 10, 17,

Lactic acid,
    and cool-down, 104,
    and muscle development, 74,
    and training to failure, 30, 43,
    definition and current hypotheses, 5, 6,
    fatigue acid, 5, 6,
    oxygen's impact, 5, 6,
    see also failure, muscular exhaustion,
    see also fatigue acid,
    see also vascularization,
    sprinter versus jogger, 5,

Lifting technique,
    bodybuilder, 107-108,
    competitive weight lifter, 107,
    controlled momentum for maximum vascularization, 108,

Lifting to failure,
    definition, 73-74,
    key to strength and vascularisation, 73,
    lactic acid buildup, 74,
    maximum intensity, 74,
    see also muscular exhaustion,
    see also principle of moderation,
    spotting technique and objectives, 74,

Lipids,
    and cardiovascular disease, 57,
    definition, 53,
    diet and behaviour guidelines, 57-58,
    dietary cholesterol, 54-55,
    fat composition, 55,
    functions, 53,
    lipoproteins, 54,
    monounsaturated fats, 56,
    polyunsaturated fats, 56,
    saturated fat, 56,
    source, 53,
    trans fat, 57,
    triglycerides, 55,

Long-term adherence,
    athletic ability, 128,
    being properly informed, xv,
    exercising while at work, 128
    how to maintain, xiv, xv,
    motivation, 127,
    see also diminishing returns,
    why crucial, xiv,
    working excessively, 127,

Lumen,
    lumen size and atherosclerosis, 9,
    lumen size and blood pressure, 9, 15
    see also arteries,

Mean arterial pressure,
    calculating formula, 35,
    definition, 35,
    rationale, 35,
    see also diastolic pressure,
    see also systolic pressure,
    systolic versus diastolic pressure, 35,

Measuring your resting blood pressure,
    average of multiple readings and reliability, 34,
    how taken, 34,
    why multiple readings, xv, 34,

Mesomorphic build,
 and BMI, 40,
 definition, 40,

Metabolic needs,
 and capillary density, 14, 23,
 and heart and aortic contractions, 8,
 and increased resistance, 8,
 of a vascularised organ, 14, 16,
 see also atherosclerosis,
 see also metabolism,
 see also vascularisation,

Metabolism,
 definition, 67,
 see also resting metabolic rate, RMR,

Metabolite,
 definition, 5,
 organ's involuntary response to, 5,
 rate of production, 5,
 see also metabolic needs,
 see also metabolism,
 sprinter versus jogger, 5,
 the metabolite carbon dioxide, 5,
 the metabolite lactic acid, 5, 6, 104,

Milking action,
 definition, 16,
 and well-functioning muscles, 16,
 and exertion-induced blood pressure, 43,

Mitochondrion,
 and oxygen requirement, 21,
 definition, 16,
 its function, 16,

Monitoring progress,
 five reliable tests xiv, xv, 127,
 see also heart rate,
 see also waist-weight procedure,

Motor unit,
 definition, 79,
 feedback during a lift, 80,
 finely-skilled movements, 79,
 gross motor skills, 79,
 see also muscle striations,

Multimuscle exercise,
 and bodybuilders, 108,
 and controlled momentum, 108,
 back muscles, example, 84-85,
 concurrent contractions, 77,
 consecutive contractions, 77,
 definition, 77,

Muscle mass,
 cardiovascular training and loss of muscle mass, 61,
 dieting and loss of muscle mass, 61,
 impact of weight-training on muscle mass, 61,
 increase recommended, 30, 61, 101,
 muscle mass vascularised, and blood pressure, 30,
 see also hypertrophy of skeletal muscle,
 see also insulin,
 see also waist-weight procedure,

Muscle-fat composition,
 causes of weight gain, 61-62,
 impact of cardiovascular training on muscle mass, 61,
 impact of diet alone on muscle mass, 61,
 impact of weight training on muscle mass, 61,
 monitoring muscle-fat composition, xv, 39, 61,
 questioning BMI technique, xv, 39-40,
 questioning electronic impedance instruments, 63,
 questioning skinfold techniques, xv, 40-41,

151

recommended muscle gain, 30, 61,
see also hypertrophy of skeletal muscle,
see also muscle mass
see body mass index,
see skinfold technique,
waist-hip ratio, 63,
waist-weight monitoring technique, 62,

Muscle strength,
definition, 71,
force? applied against a resistance, 71,
see also muscle tone,
see also overload principle,

Muscle striations,
alignment of striations, 79, 80-81,
attachments of origin and insertion for pectoralis major, 81,
definition and composition, 80,
direction of limb movement – pectoralis major, 80-81,
illustration: striations of the pectoralis major, 80,
insertion and origin: response to a contraction, 81,
see also insertion,
see also origin,
see also whole muscle training,

Muscle tone,
and abdominals, 101,
and strength training, 88,
definition, 88,
how maintained at rest, 88,
length of muscle versus its muscle tone, 88,
postural considerations, 88-89,
quicker response, 88,

Muscular endurance,
definition, 41, 71,
due to increased aerobic or anaerobic capacity?, 41,
factors affecting muscular endurance, 71,
mitochondrial density, 41,
slow twitch or fast twitch muscle cells?, 41,
versus cardiovascular endurance, 41, 72,

Muscular exhaustion, failure,
benefits, xiv, 40, 43,
see also failure, muscular exhaustion,

Muscular resistance,
and designing exercises, 72,
possibilities, 72,
resistance training, 72, 101,

Negative rep,
benefit, 110,
see also eccentric muscle contraction,

No pain, no gain,
build tolerance gradually to effort required for results, 48,
see also long term adherence,
see also Rocky Balboa effort,

Obesity,
BMI guidelines, 39,

Older participants,
capabilities xv, 128,

Origin of a muscle cell,
definition, 81,
role in movement, 81,

Osteoporosis,
and heavy weights, 102,
fitness benefit, xv,
its prevention, 102,

Overload principle,
    atrophy, 72,
    definition, 72,
    force used and speed of lift, 72,
    force used versus weight lifted, 72,
    strength and hypertrophy, 72,
    use in the design of exercises, 72
    what can provide resistance, 72,

Overtraining,
    cause, 76,
    recommended solution, 77,
    see adhesions,
    severe symptoms, 76,

Pacemakers,
    palliative technique, xiii,

Palliative techniques,
    limitations xiii,
    treatments for cardiovascular problems xiii,

Peripheral circulation,
    and skeletal muscles, 29,
    definition 29,
    see also core circulation,

Personal fitness program,
    general objectives, 107,
    hours required, 107,
    see also author,
    see also health-oriented fitness program,
    see also lifting technique; initial six weeks;
        principle of moderation; heart of
        the program; different angles; strict
        repetitions; rest periods; session 1;
        session 2; session 3,
    see also whole muscle training,

Perceived exertion scale,
    definition, 45,
    limitations, 45,
    valid alternative, 45,

Post exercise hypotension,
    definition, 17,
    benefits, 17

Posture,
    see also agonist,
    see also antagonist,
    see also muscle tone,

Prehypertensive blood pressure,
    and resistance to blood flow, 10,
    definition, 8,

Prime movers,
    benefit to the muscle, 88,
    definition, 87,
    role in movement, 87,
    see also agonist,
    see also multimuscle exercises,
    see also stabilizers,

Principle of moderation,
    blood supply to a muscle versus to a
        tendon, 109,
    for safety and tolerance, xv,
    see also heart of the program,
    to protect tendons, 109,

Progressive overload principle,
    definition and objectives, 72,
    for cardiovascular training, 47-49,
    for safety and tolerance, xv,
    for weight training, 72,
    new weight versus previous
        weight, 72,
    safety guidelines, 72-73,
    see also overload principle.
    see also principle of moderation,

vascularisation of larger muscles and
    blood pressure, 73,
working larger muscles versus smaller
    muscles, 73,

Proteins and amino acids,
    avoid bodybuilder consumption
        guidelines, 66-67,
    muscle cell damage by weight training, 66,
        76,
    proper diet, xv,
    why required, 66,

Public Health Agency of Canada,
    general guidelines xiii,
    limitations, xiii,
    valid alternative, xiii,

Pulse rate,
    definition, 6,
    how taken, 6,
    see also contraction pattern of the heart,

Pyramid down,
    benefits, 75,
    objective, 75,
    see also overloading,
    technique, 75,

Range of motion,
    and vascularisation, 75,
    example: pec dec flies, 75,
    objective, 75,
    test by feeling contractions, 75,

Rate of blood flow,
    purpose, 7,
    roles of heart and aorta, 8,
    see also flow rate of blood,
    see also metabolic needs,
    see also resistance to blood flow,

Red cell count,
    and cardiovascular exercises, 16,
    benefit, 16,

Recovery,
    beginning a program, 76,
    benefits of resting, 76,
    muscle cell damage and soreness, 76,
    recommendations, 76,
    see also adhesions,
    see also overtraining,

Recruiting muscle cells,
    decline bench press, 83,
    incline bench press, 83,
    multimuscle exercise, 84,
    regular bench press, 82,
    see also whole muscle training,

Reduce Blood Pressure Through Weight
    Training (title),
    and vascularisation xiv,
    medication-free lifestyle tool xiv,
    objectives, xiii-xvi,
    see also author,

Relaxation of the ventricles,
    pressure gradient, 24,
    see also contraction pattern of the heart,
    see also diastole,
    see also systole,
    see also windkessel effect
    unit of measurement, 24,
    zero ventricular pressure, 24,

Renal denervation technique,
    palliative surgical technique, xiii,

Resistance to blood flow,
    and capillary density, 23,
    and number of organs vascularised, 23,

consequences of increased resistance, 8, 10,
determinants: atherosclerosis,
    arteriosclerosis, sedentary lifestyle,
    8-10,
identical resistance of capillaries, 23,
increased resistance, reduced flow rate
    and metabolic needs, 8,
increasing the lumen diameter of arteries,
    15,
measuring the overall resistance R/n of
    an organ, 23,
see also flow rate of blood,
see also rate of blood flow,
weight training and peripheral resistance,
    30,

Resistance to muscle-initiated movement,
    definition, 72
    see also overload principle,

Resting metabolic rate (RMR),
    and age, 67,
    and body fat, 67,
    and capillary density, 14, 23,
    benefit of raising RMR, 67,
    definition, 67,
    how to raise RMR, 67,
    muscle versus fat tissue, 30, 67,
    see also metabolism,

Resting blood pressure,
    and appropriate physical activity, 33,
    and overtraining, 102,
    as a baseline reference value, 33-34,
    correlation with resting pulse rate, 45,
    definition, 8,
    how taken, 34,
    response to metabolite levels, 3,
    see also blood pressure,
    see also monitoring progress,
    why take it, 10, 34,

Resting diastolic pressure,
    and appropriate physical activity, 33,
    see also resting blood pressure,

Resting pulse rate,
    and exercise intensity (including weight
        training), 44,
    and marathon running, 6,
    and resting blood pressure, 6, 11, 44,
    as a baseline reference value, 6,
    cardiovascular health indicator, 6, 7,
    definition, 6,
    how taken and how often, 6,
    response to cardiovascular activity, 6,
    see also monitoring progress,

Resting systolic pressure,
    and appropriate physical activity, 33,
    see also resting blood pressure,

Rest periods,
    pattern followed during personal fitness
        program, 110-111,

Rocky Balboa effort,
    why unacceptable, xiv,
    and no pain no gain, 47-48,

Sarcopenia,
    and age, 101,
    definition, 101,
    weight training for prevention, 101,

Session 1 - Monday,
    cardiovascular, 115,
    concentration and hand-eye coordination,
        115,
    exercise program for biceps and
        quadriceps, 111-115,
    frequency, once per week, 107,
    mobility and cool-down, 115,

Session 2 - Wednesday,
    cardiovascular, 121,
    concentration and hand-eye coordination, 121,
    exercise program for triceps and back, 116-120,
    frequency, once per week, 107,
    mobility and cool-down, 121,

Session 3 - Friday,
    cardiovascular, 125,
    concentration and hand-eye coordination, 126,
    exercise program for shoulders and chest, 122-125,
    frequency, once per week, 107,
    mobility and cool-down, 126,

Skinfold technique,
    and muscle-fat composition, 39,
    correlates with fat content only, 39,
    limitations, 40,
    procedure and calculation, 40,
    site-specificity of exercise for fat reduction, 41,
    versus waist-weight method, xv, 39, 61-63,
    waist measurement adequate, 41,

Specificity of weight training,
    and isometric training, 74,
    definition, 74,
    role in designing exercises, 74, 89,
    see also whole muscle training,

Sports-oriented program,
    choice of exercises, 97,
    initial analysis: gymnast – wrester – marathon runner – football lineman – quarterback – bodybuilder, 96-97,
    objectives, 95-96,
    practical component of training, 97,

Stabilizers,
    benefit from weight training? , 88,
    definition, 87,
    example: upper and lower back muscles during bicep curls, 87,
    role in movement, 87,
    see also multimuscle exercises,
    see also prime movers,

Starting weights,
    best approach, 42,
    current approach, 42,
    definition, 42,
    safety concerns, 42,

Strength training,
    agonist versus antagonist, 102,
    benefits: calories burnt, resting metabolic rate, functionality, insulin resistance, lowering blood pressure, 101,
    bone development, 102,
    calcium metabolism, 101-102,
    isometric versus isotonic training, 74,
    safety considerations, 73,
    see also lifting to failure,
    see also muscle strength,
    see also muscular endurance,
    see also pyramid down,
    see also range of motion,
    see also sarcopenia,
    see also the overload principle,
    see also the principle of moderation,
    see also the progressive overload principle,
    see also whole muscle training,
    strength development, 101-102,
    term "lifting heavy weight" is relative, xiv, 102,

Stretching,
    for elasticity (flexibility), 100,
    how often, 100,

safety considerations, 100,
technique, 100,
to offset postural imbalances, 100,
warm-up component, 100,

Strict repetitions,
definition, 110,
purpose, 110,
weight lifted, 110,

Stroke,
cause, 10,
damaged brain cells do not heal, 10,
massive stroke; some symptoms, xvii,

Swiss exercise balls,
limitations, 46,
objectives, 46,
see faddish fitness programs,
wobbly versus stable surface, 46,

Systolic blood pressure,
and capillary density, 14, 30, 31, 33,
and cardiovascular training, xiv, 29,
and detraining, 77,
and increased resistance to blood flow, 10,
definition, and ratio form expression, 8,
neurogenic and biochemical controls, 26,
pre-hypertensive and hypertensive levels, 8, 10,
response to stress, 34,
role of the left ventricle, 24-26,
see also windkessel effect,
versus diastolic (MAP), 35,
without the aorta's contribution, 8,

Systole,
calcium-releasing mechanism, 24,
definition, 24,
see also contraction pattern of the heart,
see also windkessel effect,
zero ventricular pressure, 24,

Thrombolytic therapy (clot-busting drugs),
palliative medication technique, xiii,

Tolerance,
and older participants, xv,
and weight training, 49,
for physical discomfort, at a safe and reasonable pace, xv,
limitations of no pain, no gain approach, 47-48,
pace of desired physical changes, 48,
sample graduated approach, 48,
see also progressive overload principle,

Topping up the ventricles,
during diastole, 24,

Training effect,
see also detraining effect,
vascularization 13-17,

Triceps,
anatomy, 108,
see also antagonist,

Unidirectional valves,
description and function, 5, 16,
see also veins,

Vascularization,
benefits of the effectuated changes, 14-15, 23-24,
changes effectuated, 13-17, 19,
definition, 13, 16,
see capillary density, through cardiovascular training, xiv, 13,
through weight training xiv,

Vascularized muscle mass,
and microcirculatory blood volume, 21,
increasing capillary density, 20-21,

oxygen requirement, 19-20,
research results, 19-21,
see also muscle mass,

Vasoconstrict,
arterioles, 5,
purpose, 5,

Vasodilate,
arterioles, 5,
purpose, 5,

Veins,
and capillary density, 13,
and milking action, 16, 43,
compliance 5,
description and function, 3, 5, 13,
see also blood,
see also unidirectional valves,

Ventricles,
illustration, 7,
see also systole,
see also systolic pressure,
see also windkessel effect,
thickness of left ventricular wall, 7,

Visceral fat,
and fatty acids, 65,
and waistline, 65,
description, 65,
dieting considerations, 66,
Dr. Yang, appetite and NPY, 66,
limitations of exercise in reducing visceral fat, 65-66,
see also dieting,
why dangerous, 65,

Waist-hip ratio,
and cardiovascular disease, 63,
ideal waist size, 62,
procedure and measurement, 40,
see also waist-weight procedure,
validity versus BMI, 40,

Waist-weight procedure,
see also monitoring progress,
to monitor muscle-fat composition, 62,
versus BMI and skinfold techniques, xv, 39,
versus electronic impedance measurements, 63,
waist-hip ratio for ideal waist size, 63,

Warm-up,
for safety: muscle and tendon elasticity, 100,
objective, 100,
see also cool-down,
see also crunches,
see also health-oriented fitness program,
stretching technique, 100,

Watered-down programs,
effectiveness, xv,
see also older participants,

Weight-training,
additional benefits, 30,
and blood pressure xiv,
and cardiovascular health, 29-30,
and vascularization of skeletal muscle xiv,
damage to muscle cells, 66, 76,
impact on blood pressure versus cardio, 30,
intensity required, 30,
muscle hypertrophy and blood pressure, 31,
need for proteins and amino acids, 66,
see also breathing,
see also hypertrophy of skeletal muscle,
impact on cholesterol levels, 67,
see also strength training
see whole muscle training,

term heavy weight is relative, xiv, 102,
versus bodybuilding xiv,
weight training principles, chapter 12,

Whole muscle training,
action to be overloaded, 82, 83, 84,
and vascularisation, 79,
back muscle to illustrate multimuscle training, 84-85,
brain recruitment of muscle cells, 82, 84,
critical, xv,
regular, decline and incline bench press to train the whole pectoralis major, 81-84,
role of muscle fiber alignment in designing exercises , 80,
see motor units,
see muscle striations,

Windkessel effect,
impact on blood pressure, 8, 24-26,
phases involved including the aortic recoil, 25-26,
purpose, 8, 26,
role of neurogenic and feedback mechanisms, 26,
see also blood pressure,
see also diastolic pressure,
see also systolic pressure

Made in the USA
Charleston, SC
20 July 2014